Psychology
ADHD
KUT

618.92/KUT

3206166

P9-CCZ-300

Praise for the first edition

"A heart-gladdening investigation into the world of adolescents caught in the syndrome mix, and how to identify symptoms, understand the causes and embark on treatments for each condition. Kutscher…has written an exemplary introductory guide through the baffling worlds of ADHD, learning disability, the autistic spectrum, anxiety, obsessive compulsive disorder, tics, depression, bipolar, oppositional defiant disorder, and central auditory processing disorder. Why all these under one cover? Because so often kids come with multiple issues, which impinge upon and amplify one another. After Kutscher finishes explaining what is known about the causes of the disorders, he unveils concrete strategies and high-yield recommendations on how to proceed. Like a good doctor, his first piece of advice is to do no harm: you are the lifeline for your child or charge, so you must be positive and calm, and you must not nag, lecture, argue, or offer untimely advice. You must pursue a course conducive to the circumstances. And Kutscher offers a spectrum of approaches that are practical and executable. He also tackles the available pharmacopoeia, and he has plenty of suggested resources for further reading… A sparkling, granite-strong steppingstone from which to launch further investigations into the conditions Kutscher covers, though, given its myriad hands-on recommendations, this guide may be an end in itself."

—*Kirkus Reports*

"For 18 years, Kutscher…has been diagnosing often co-existing neuropsychiatric disorders like attention deficit hyperactivity disorder, autistic spectrum disorders, learning difficulties, and bipolar disorder. His accessible and comprehensive guide covers the general principles of diagnosis and treatment of those disorders in children; individual chapters on each condition elucidate causes, symptoms, interactions between conditions, and treatments. Parents and professionals alike will find the behavioral strategies, case vignettes, and practical tips particularly helpful… As the first book to cover such a wide range of disorders for lay readers, this is highly recommended for public libraries with special-needs parenting sections."

—*Library Journal*

Barclay Public Library
220 South Main Street
PO Box 349
Warrensburg, IL 62573

"*Kids in the Syndrome Mix* is an interesting, extremely well-written book. Easy to read, it is a concise guide to the whole range of neuro-behavioral disorders in children. From detection of the problem it also gives good advice on coping, managing, and treatment for these various disorders. Invaluable help for families, teachers, etc. who have a child affected in this way... It is certainly the best in its field."

—*No Panic*

"Dr. Kutscher not only makes difficult information easier to understand, but does it with a depth of understanding and compassion that is unique in the field. His examples are true to life and his strategies concrete and applicable in everyday life. I would strongly recommend this book to be on any teacher's reading list and a guide for parents dealing with children with special challenges. If I had my wish I would make it mandatory reading for every teacher coming out of teacher's college. I will be recommending it frequently."

—*Heidi Bernhardt, Director, ADRN (Attention Deficit Research Network), Toronto, Canada*

"This is a groundbreaking, terrific, thoroughly researched, and brilliantly written, interpretive treatise of oft-misunderstood, frequently diagnosed disorders with numerous interventions provided by a literary genius."

—*Gayle M. Bell, EdS, Educational Specialist, Coeur d'Alene, ID, US*

"While recognizing and validating the frustration that parents and teachers may experience on a daily basis when dealing with a dysregulated child, Dr. Kutscher skillfully manages to create both empathy for the child and a positive outlook for the difference informed and caring parents and teachers can make... I think that this book would serve as a useful quick guide for teachers as part of their school's special needs library... It's wonderful to have one book I can recommend to parents so that they can find helpful information on all of their child's conditions in one place."

—*Leslie Packer, PhD, specialist in Tourette's Syndrome, consulting psychologist to school districts, and clinician in private practice*

KIDS IN THE SYNDROME MIX OF ADHD, LD, AUTISM SPECTRUM, TOURETTE'S, ANXIETY, AND MORE!

2ND EDITION

by the same author

ADHD
Living without Brakes
Martin L. Kutscher MD
Illustrated by Douglas Puder MD
ISBN 978 1 84310 873 3 (hardback)
ISBN 978 1 84905 816 2 (paperback)
eISBN 978 1 84642 769 5

Children with Seizures
A Guide for Parents, Teachers, and Other Professionals
Martin L. Kutscher MD
Foreword by Gregory L. Holmes MD
Part of the *JKP Essentials* series
ISBN 978 1 84310 823 8
eISBN 978 1 84642 490 8

of related interest

The Complete Guide to Asperger's Syndrome
Tony Attwood
ISBN 978 1 84310 495 7 (hardback)
ISBN 978 1 84310 669 2 (paperback)
eISBN 978 1 84642 559 2

Tics and Tourette Syndrome
A Handbook for Parents and Professionals
Uttom Chowdhury
ISBN 978 1 84310 203 8
eISBN 978 1 84642 006 1

Asperger Syndrome
What Teachers Need to Know
2nd Edition
Matt Winter
With Clare Lawrence
ISBN 978 1 84905 203 0
eISBN 978 0 85700 430 7

All Cats Have Asperger Syndrome
Kathy Hoopmann
ISBN 978 1 84310 481 0

KIDS IN THE SYNDROME MIX OF
ADHD, LD, AUTISM SPECTRUM, TOURETTE'S, ANXIETY, AND MORE!

2ND EDITION

The one-stop guide for parents,
teachers, and other professionals

Martin L. Kutscher, MD
With contributions from Tony Attwood, PhD
and Robert R. Wolff, MD

Jessica Kingsley *Publishers*
London and Philadelphia

Disclaimer: The information in this book does not constitute medical advice, which can only be given by direct discussion between patients and their doctors. Like most areas of information, knowledge about mental health issues is likely to change over time. The views of cited references do not necessarily represent the views of the authors. Some of the common medication uses described in this text are not currently FDA approved.

Figure 3.1 (p.61) uses illustrations kindly provided by Taylor Vittora Rino.

This edition first published in 2014
by Jessica Kingsley Publishers
73 Collier Street
London N1 9BE, UK
and
400 Market Street, Suite 400
Philadelphia, PA 19106, USA

www.jkp.com

First edition published in 2005 by Jessica Kingsley Publishers

Copyright © Martin L. Kutscher 2014
Chapter 6 copyright © Tony Attwood 2014

All rights reserved. No part of this publication may be reproduced in any material form (including photocopying or storing it in any medium by electronic means and whether or not transiently or incidentally to some other use of this publication) without the written permission of the copyright owner except in accordance with the provisions of the Copyright, Designs and Patents Act 1988 or under the terms of a licence issued by the Copyright Licensing Agency Ltd, Saffron House, 6–10 Kirby Street, London EC1N 8TS. Applications for the copyright owner's written permission to reproduce any part of this publication should be addressed to the publisher.

Warning: The doing of an unauthorised act in relation to a copyright work may result in both a civil claim for damages and criminal prosecution.

Library of Congress Cataloging in Publication Data
Kutscher, Martin L.
  Kids in the syndrome mix of ADHD, LD, autism spectrum, Tourette's, anxiety and more! : the one stop guide for parents, teachers and other professionals / Martin L. Kutscher ; with contributions from Tony Attwood and Robert R. Wolff, MD. -- 2nd edition.
    pages cm
  Includes bibliographical references and index.
  ISBN 978-1-84905-967-1 (alk. paper)
  1. Behavior disorders in children. 2. Attention-deficit hyperactivity disorder. 3. Learning disabled children. 4. Tourette syndrome in children. 5. Manic-depressive illness in children. 6. Child psychopathology. 7. Asperger's syndrome. 8. Autism in children. I. Attwood, Tony. II. Wolff, Robert R. III. Title.
  RJ506.B44K88 2014
  618.92'858832--dc23

                            2013040239

British Library Cataloguing in Publication Data
A CIP catalogue record for this book is available from the British Library

ISBN 978 1 84905 967 1
eISBN 978 0 85700 882 4

Printed and bound in the United States

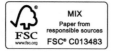

To my wife, whose constant attention to our family continues to amaze me.

To my children, whose very existence is a miracle.

To the mothers of my patients, who give unconditional love to their children.

And to my patients, who didn't choose to have the problems that they cope with daily.

Contents

Introduction 11

Chapter 1   Read this Chapter! General Principles
of Diagnosis 17

Chapter 2   Read this Chapter! General Principles
of Treatment 27

Chapter 3   Attention Deficit Hyperactivity Disorder 53

Chapter 4   Specific Learning Disorders (LDs) 81
Robert R. Wolff, MD and Martin L. Kutscher, MD

Chapter 5   Autism Spectrum Disorder (ASD): An Overview. 111

Chapter 6   Autism Spectrum Disorder, Level 1 (Asperger's
Syndrome) and its Treatment. 137
Tony Attwood, PhD

Chapter 7   Anxiety and Obsessive-Compulsive Disorders . . . 171

Chapter 8   Sensory Integration Dysfunction (SID or SPD) . . 183
Martin L. Kutscher, MD with Joelle Glick

Chapter 9   Tics and Tourette's 197

Chapter 10   Depression 207

Chapter 11   Bipolar Disorder 219

Chapter 12   Oppositional Defiant Disorder (ODD) and
Intermittent Explosive Disorder 231

Chapter 13   Central Auditory Processing Disorders (CAPDs) . 241

Chapter 14   Medications 253

APPENDIX 1   BEHAVIORAL CHECKLIST   281

APPENDIX 2   QUICK QUIZ ON EXECUTIVE FUNCTION   285

APPENDIX 3   DEALING WITH INSOMNIA: SLEEP HYGIENE   289

APPENDIX 4   FURTHER READING   291

REFERENCES   301

ABOUT THE AUTHORS   307

SUBJECT INDEX   309

AUTHOR INDEX   317

Introduction

Why this book?

There are kids out there who need help. They have attention deficit hyperactivity disorder (ADHD), or learning disabilities (LDs), or tics, or autism spectrum disorder, or depression, or any combination of many problems. We want to assist, but how? There is a lot to learn about what we shall call the "syndrome mix."

There are superb books that cover each of these topics in detail, and I encourage you to consult the Further Reading section (Appendix 4) for suggestions. However, this updated edition has been developed for the following reasons:

- We need one book that covers multiple problems in a single place, because that's the way so many kids come: multiple issues in a single child. Co-occurrence of several difficulties is the norm, not the exception. If a child has one condition (such as learning disabilities or anxiety), he has a 40% chance of having at least one other mental disorder (CDC 2013).

- What parent, teacher, or therapist has time to read about all those conditions from multiple books? I have had parents tell me, "If our home was calm enough for me to find time to read all of those books you suggested, then I would not have needed them in the first place." Teachers and other professionals are busy, too. (I know. I have the pleasure to be married to a high school teacher.)

- Even more problematic, these excellent books can have an overwhelming number of suggestions to be implemented—leading all too frequently to none of them being used.

- The goal of this book, then, is to provide the needed information in a format that will:

  ◦ cover multiple neuropsychiatric conditions in one text, striving to show how these syndromes frequently mix together in the same child

  ◦ present a brief, informal distillation of crux material in a realistic but upbeat format. We explain the cause, symptoms, and treatment of each problem. Excess verbiage is shunned. A little humor along the way will help keep our perspective

  ◦ provide a small number of high-yield recommendations. If even these few suggestions are implemented, there will be significant effect. The book does not attempt to make the reader into full-clad special education teachers or psychiatrists.

- This second edition has been updated to conform to the new *Diagnostic and Statistical Manual of Mental Disorders*, version 5 (DSM-5) of the American Psychiatric Association released in 2013. The DSM is the de facto "official" American classification of mental disorders. Important changes in DSM terminology are presented, along with the earlier terms they replace. However, we will not over-emphasize the DSM, since, as its name actually states, it is a diagnostic and (research) statistical tool. The criteria it sets out are of more use to researchers and to your doctors than to parents, for whom understanding the symptoms and their treatment is more helpful. For example, knowing that a DSM-5 criterion for ADHD is at least partial onset before age 12 does little to help parents care for their child's impulsivity. Plus, the fact that DSM is already up to version 5 should lay to rest any thought that it is an indisputable "bible."

- This second edition also brings updated insights into the etiology and treatments of the conditions of the syndrome mix.

The magnitude of the problems: as measured by statistics

The US CDC (Centers for Disease Control) data reveals that in any given year between 13% and 20% of US children will experience a mental disorder. Specific rates for some of these conditions are:

- ADHD: 6.8%

- behavioral or conduct problem: 3.5%

- anxiety: 3.0%

- depression: 2.1%

- autism spectrum disorders: 1.1%

- Tourette's syndrome: 0.2%

- Suicide is the second leading cause of death of children of 12–17 years of age.

(CDC 2013)

Other research indicates the following:

- Despite the fact that nearly one-fifth of children have a mental illness, only one-fifth of these children receive treatment.

- There is an eight to ten year gap between a child's onset of symptoms and his being brought to the attention of a health professional.

(Houston 2013)

The magnitude of the problems:
as measured in human terms

But what is the magnitude of the problem in human, emotional terms? Nothing less is at stake than our child's sense of self-worth, confidence, resiliency, and happiness. And, with that, follows our own happiness. After all, it's been said that a parent is only as happy as his least happy child. Sometimes, the challenge of a special needs child binds parents together and sometimes it splits them apart. Sometimes, the challenge leads to parental fulfillment and growth and sometimes it leads to bitter resentment. Hopefully, the knowledge and understanding that comes from this book will help you and your family on your journey and its detours. It's going to be quite a trip, but you'll make it. After all, you have no other choice.

Who is this book for?

This book is intended for:

- parents and other relatives

- teachers

- learning specialists

- psychologists and physicians

- social workers and counselors

- speech, occupational, and physical therapists

- anyone else who comes into contact with these kids.

How can one book apply to so many groups? Well, aren't all of these people on the same team, with the shared goal of helping the same child? Don't all of these groups need to understand what is happening in the multiple spheres of the child's life at home, school, and therapy? Don't they all need to know about the underpinnings of a large variety of problems in the syndrome mix? Indeed, don't all groups need trained eyes in order to make and share appropriate observations and suggestions?

How to use this book

Everyone initially should read the first two chapters. These cover the general principles of diagnosis and treatment that apply to virtually all conditions. Grouping these principles together at the front allows us to avoid repeating them in each chapter.

Next, you can pick out the chapters that relate to your specific, immediate needs. Hopefully, you can also read the symptom sections of all of the chapters. Unless we know something about the full range of conditions in the syndrome mix, we risk pigeonholing everyone into those diagnoses that we do know about, or we may stop looking for additional ones.

At the end of the book, there is a chapter on medication, a behavioral checklist, suggestions for sleep hygiene, and recommended further reading. Some of the chapters contain links to the author's website www.pediatricneurology.com. These links provide multimedia simulations that supplement the text.

Good luck with your kids! You are their lifeline. Failure is not an option.

CHAPTER 1

Read this Chapter!
General Principles of Diagnosis

"How am I supposed to figure out what the problem is? I'm not a doctor."

The "syndrome mix"

Conditions of the "syndrome mix"
typically occur in clusters

Start with a real, live child—a kid with feelings, needs, and hopes. Mix in a double helping of attention deficit hyperactivity disorder (ADHD), a touch of Tourette's, and a dash of dysgraphia. Stir gently. That's one possible "syndrome mix" that a child, parent, and teacher, and other professionals, may be given. That's what they have to deal with.

Who says that kids have just one problem? Multiple issues frequently cluster together in any combination. Common members of the syndrome mix include:

- ADHD

- learning disability (LD)

- autism spectrum disorder

- anxiety/obsessive-compulsive disorder (OCD)

- Tourette's syndrome

- depression

- bipolar disorder

- oppositional defiant disorder

- central auditory processing disorder

- sensory integration dysfunction.

If a child has any one of the problems out of the syndrome mix, there is a very significant chance of one or more of the other problems also occurring. As an example, two-thirds of children with ADHD have at least one of these other "co-morbidities," and one-third of children with ADHD have at least two of them (Larson *et al.* 2011). Alternatively, the vast majority of children with Tourette's syndrome who make it to a referral center also have co-occurring anxiety/OCD and ADHD.

Not only does a child tend to be born with multiple issues, but the issues also may *exacerbate* each other. For example, a child may innately have both ADHD and learning disabilities, but then the poor attention span makes it harder to learn, while the difficulty learning makes it harder to concentrate. The mix of syndromes keeps exacerbating itself.

Similarly, the problems can *imitate* each other. For example, a child constantly mulling over her anxieties can look distracted, and this behavior can be confused with ADHD.

In addition, often the stressed child will find himself in a stressed home or school environment. It is true that the stressful environment may have been caused by the child, but the end result is that the child now finds himself having to deal with stressed-out adults—the last ingredient the child needs!

Also, many of the neuropsychiatric conditions run in families. Thus, the child may find herself coping with parents, teachers, and therapists with their own inborn problems. Indeed, while considering possible titles for this book, my wife kind-heartedly suggested, "What Did You Think Would Happen When You Married Your Spouse?"

Conditions of the "syndrome mix" are not all or nothing

Importantly, for each area of difficulty, there is a gradient of severity. We need to separate whether it is a "problem" (i.e., significantly impacts the quality of a child's life and merits significant intervention) or a "quirk" (i.e., an unusual feature causing less impairment). Even if an issue does not rise to criteria for a "problem" status, it might still benefit from being addressed. Dr. John Ratey, a noted psychiatrist, refers to these low-grade issues as "shadow syndromes" (Ratey and Johnson 1998).

One reason, then, that parents and teachers may have trouble figuring out what *the* problem is that there is typically more than one, each occurring with its own degree of intensity.

First signs

When you think about it, psychologists, therapists, neurologists, and psychiatrists do not stand on the street corner and randomly pick children to evaluate. Rather, the kids are all sent there because other people have noticed a problem. Those people are the ones on the frontline: the parents and the teachers. They may not know *what* the problem is, but these caregivers are the first to diagnose that there *is* a problem. Like it or not, the whole system depends on these first-responders. This chapter will help you feel more comfortable filling the role you have already been given.

No child's problem is diagnosed on the basis of one piece of information. Over time, multiple observers all become increasingly aware that there is some problem. The concerns typically brew over several years, until someone finally gets sufficiently frustrated to say, "Hey, there's a pattern here. Something is up!" What observations, then, typically lead to a diagnosis?

Parents' observations

No one knows a child like the parents. Mothers typically have nagging (or sometimes blatant) concerns long before anyone else will listen. Mothers are the ones who keep seeing and hearing the same things. They are the ones with whom the child confides. They typically bear the brunt of the child's frustrations.

If parents see that something is wrong, they are typically right. After all, most parents are not interested in "making up" problems for their children. Would parents schedule a school meeting or a doctor's appointment just for the experience of falsely declaring to the world that their child is not thriving? No—if a parent is concerned, then there *is* usually an issue. That is not to say, though, that the parents have necessarily correctly identified *what* the problem is, or *who* is responsible for fixing it—just that there *is* a problem.

Teachers' observations

Teachers are incredibly valuable in the identification of a child's difficulties, for multiple reasons.

- They spend a great deal of time with the child, second only to the parents.

- They have had contact with many other children over time, helping them to establish a basis of "typical."

- They have ongoing typical "control" of children in the class. They can see which child is different from all of the others in the same classroom.

- If a teacher is experiencing a problem with a child, then, by definition, there is a problem.

- When report card comments are read in sequence, there is usually significant conformity over the years. This pattern attests that the difficulty is with a particular child, rather than a particular teacher–student match.

In order to find the teachers' concerns, though, we must be aware that the issues are frequently masked underneath otherwise positive comments. The teacher tries not to be too negative, especially if the child is perceived as kind, cute, smart, or hard working. For example, he might say, "Jill can do such amazing work when she puts her mind to it!" On the surface, it's a positive comment about Jill's intelligence. The subtext, though, is that Jill is not always on task.

In addition to written comments, checklists can also be helpful. Anyone can use the Behavioral Checklist (see Appendix 1). For ADHD evaluations, guidance counselors or the doctor can provide a similar quick-rating scale.

Here are the take-home messages for teachers:

- Although the teachers' role may not be to make a specific diagnosis, their input is key to the process. Teacher feedback is the basis for diagnosing any school-related problem.

- Detailed written teacher comments allow for "hidden messages" to come through, and provide the doctor with objective information. Ask the teachers to write a few paragraphs answering: "How is Johnny doing?" Comments may be supplemented with check-off forms.

- When a teacher identifies a problem, there usually is one. However, the teacher may be less accurate at identifying the true underlying *cause* of the difficulty.

- Teachers might seek the guidance of their school professionals (psychologists, guidance counselors, etc.) before broaching the idea of seeking a doctor's guidance with the parents.

Common pitfalls

If you find yourself saying any of the following, be very cautious. They are red flags of misinterpreting the child's behaviors.

- *"He's lazy."* You'll notice that "lazy" is not listed in this or any textbook as a possible diagnosis. I've yet to meet a child who woke up one morning and had the following silent conversation: "Hmm. I wonder if I should try my best today, get good grades, and be praised? Or, maybe I should deliberately blow off my work and get punished?

Oh, the latter choice should be fun!" Yes, by the time an undiagnosed teen gets to high school, the child may indeed have been beaten down so often that he has given up. However, if we look back over the person's history, we usually find a young child bouncing with energy. Somewhere along the way, he's learned to give up.

- *"He's so unprepared. He obviously does not care."* As we will see later, disorganization is a major part of ADHD and executive dysfunction.

- *"She only does it when she is interested."* All of us do better when we are interested. The question is, "What is going on that she can't do it at all unless the task is totally intriguing?"

- *"She'd be better at it if she just showed more interest."* No, it's probably the other way round, i.e., she'd be more interested in it if she were better at it. A child who is a poor reader will avoid the task. I doubt she ever said to herself, "Let's avoid reading until I get really bad at it."

- *"He is inconsistent. I've seen him do it, sometimes."* Just because a child has occasionally done something right, it does not mean we should hold it against him forever.

- *"She is just a social butterfly."* Boys tend to be labelled "hyper," whereas girls get called "social." True, it may be developmentally appropriate to be social; but is the girl really more interested in what her friend ate for breakfast than in learning her schoolwork, or is there some other problem? Inattentive ADHD (especially in girls) is harder to diagnose—but no less real—than ADHD with hyperactivity-impulsivity.

- *"I don't know if there is a problem. I'm just the teacher/parent."* As we've seen, there is no one else like the teacher and parent to identify the child who is having some problem.

Formal evaluation

Psycho-educational testing

If the need for potential significant intervention arises, eventually the child might be given a "psycho-educational evaluation." This consists of a detailed series of tests.

- Psychological tests (indicating a child's *potential*), including the WISC-IV (Wechsler Intelligence Scale for Children-IV)—commonly referred to as the "IQ" (intelligence quotient) test.

- Educational tests (indicating a child's *academic achievement* in areas like reading or math level), such as the Woodcock-Johnson or WIAT (Wechsler Individual Achievement Test).

The report prepared by the tester usually includes an explanation of these tests and their significance. A full child study team evaluation may also include reports from social work, speech and language, occupational therapy (for fine motor, handwriting, and sensory integration), physical therapy (for gross motor), neurology, or psychiatry. Anyone—parent or teacher—can request an evaluation by the school district's team, which should be done in a timely fashion.

The medical doctor's evaluation

What happens if the child gets sent to the medical doctor to be diagnosed? Nothing magical happens there that allows us to observe things not noted by parents and teachers over the years. In fact, the medical office is a poor place to observe a child's natural behavior. Let's take the case of a child presenting for an ADHD evaluation. One of the treatments for ADHD is a structured one-to-one situation with frequent, novel stimuli—just what occurs in the doctor's office. Thus, trying to make the diagnosis of ADHD is difficult while the child is in what should be a therapeutic setting. This is a point of confusion for many professionals, leading to the all too frequent, "I don't see anything wrong with your child." In addition, many problems such as poor foresight and organization need the laboratory of actual life over many months to be detected. Only caregivers outside of the doctor's office can make such long-term observations.

What do experienced doctors do? In addition to their own observations, they rely on real-world observations by those people who care extensively for the child: the parents and the teachers. In other words, we examine and talk to the kids; but mostly we talk to the parents, read the teacher reports, and read any testing that has been done. We try to fit all of the years of observed information into a pattern, and derive one or more diagnoses. If the medical/neurological history and physical exam suggest the need, we may sometimes perform blood tests, electroencephalograms, etc.

What accommodations should you make for your child?

Armed with all of the data, everyone gets together for the big day: teachers, guidance counselors, school evaluators, administration, advocates, and parents. This team hopefully reaches an accord as to the appropriate diagnosis and treatments.

Each country and state has its own set of laws regarding appropriate formal accommodations, and readers are advised to discuss these procedures with their local school program director. Readers can find information about terms such as "504" and "IDEA" at www.ldonline.org and www.wrightslaw.com.

This book, though, focuses on common-sense accommodations. These accommodations are not necessarily "mandated," but can be implemented by an appropriately helpful teacher/school. Many of them would be helpful to all students, not just those with special needs. Common-sense accommodations might include educating teachers about the child's diagnosis, and checking that the child really understands directions, preferential seating, etc.

Summary

The goal of helping each child to achieve her potential requires the cooperation and mutual respect of the parents, teachers, and school administrators. Parents and teachers typically have quite good insight into detecting, over time, that there is *some problem*. In order to determine *which problem(s)* exist, the diagnostician depends upon the observations of those people who devote so much of their time to the children. Sorting out the syndrome mix can be difficult, since multiple problems can be born into the same child, can occur in varying degrees of severity, can mimic each other, and can worsen each other.

CHAPTER 2

Read this Chapter!
General Principles of Treatment

A child with special needs and temperament has been entrusted to your care. If you are going to maximize the child's potential—and keep your sanity at the same time—you will need to adopt certain mindsets and strategies.

Congratulations! You've been selected to help a child in need—a role you may or may not have volunteered for, but which nonetheless represents an opportunity for growth for you and the child. The following general treatment guidelines apply to most kids with any of the syndromes in this book. We'll start with techniques for adjusting your own mindset, move on to understanding the child's mindset, and then discuss how to change the child's behavior. You don't need any formal classification or diagnosis to adopt these strategies. Specific additional guidelines for each condition are given in subsequent chapters.

Adjusting your own mindset

☐ *Accept your child.* Children who feel accepted, celebrated and secure in their relationships are free to explore, thrive, and even be more cooperative. As Brooks and Goldstein write in *Raising Resilient Children* (2001, p.12), "accepting children for who they are and appreciating their different temperaments does not mean that we excuse inappropriate, unacceptable behavior, but rather that we understand this behavior and help to change it in a manner that does not erode a child's self-esteem and sense of dignity." The rest of this book is designed to help you do just that.

☐ *Remember: "The thing I like about you best…is that you like me."* This quote from the cartoon character Ziggy applies to many human relationships, but is particularly important for kids who find themselves suddenly zapped from all angles— even from inside their own brain. Ed Hallowell and Peter Jensen (2008, p.7) put it this way, "These are the kids who need your love the most, because they get it elsewhere the least… A parent ought to be a child's first and greatest fan." If you really like the child, he is more prone to like you back.

☐ *Don't take the difficult behaviors as personal affronts.* The answer to the question "Why can't he be like all of the other children?" is that he can't—at least not yet. It isn't personal. You just happen to be the person in the room. Always remember that there is a real, live, feeling child underneath all of those problems.

It may also help to remember that the person who suffers most from these behaviors is usually the child himself. These children "shoot *themselves* in the foot" just as often as they bother anyone else. What further evidence could we have that these problems are not fully within their control?

☐ *Adopt a "disability outlook."* You do not have a standard child. You can view the issue as a wonderful uniqueness in the child, or you can view the issue as a disability. Or you can view it as both. The perspective of "standard," though, is not an option.

Dr. Russell Barkley, a leading psychologist in the field of attention deficit hyperactivity disorder (ADHD), urges caregivers to incorporate a "disability outlook" (Barkley 2013, p.166). A disability outlook is not as much "fun" as just considering these kids as unique individuals with special traits. However, it points the way for caregivers to see themselves as "therapists" for their problematic child—not as victims of him.

It may be difficult to accept some of these problems as "real disabilities."

» There is no obvious physical marker for most of the conditions.

» Unlike the situation with obviously physical disabilities (such as blindness or cerebral palsy), the problems that result from neurobehavioral disabilities often get directed *at* the caregiver. The deaf child, for example, is having difficulties, but is not attacking us. Her problems evoke in us an instinct to aid her. In contrast, the child with a behavioral problem may not comply with, or may yell at, the person who is merely trying to help. In short, these children often don't seem to be asking for help in an easily lovable way. No wonder that these disabilities are harder to accept.

» To accept that some people have a physiological reason for difficulty controlling their behavior runs counter to our deep convictions about who we are. Our society feels that we are under the control of our "personality," or "will," or "soul." It is hard for us to accept that these aspects of ourselves are so heavily under the influence of neurotransmitters. Just remember: *the human brain is physically a bunch of chemicals with illusions of grandeur.*

Unless we validate the problems as true disabilities, we will dismiss the problems, and instead, blame the person for not simply taking control of them. That attitude greatly burdens the special needs person. When it was applied to her, Liane Holliday Willey (an educator/writer with Asperger's syndrome) wrote, "I was made to feel that our struggles were like lint we could pick away and toss off, if only we would make the effort to do so" (Willey 1999, p.88).

☐ *Minimize frustrations by taking a realistic look at the child you get every day.* Periodically, take stock of who is showing up in your life every day. *This* is your starting point. Not a typical child. This is what you can likely expect today. Once teachers and parents accept this starting point (which I assure you the child does not exactly want, either), it is easier not to take everything so personally. Anger on the caregiver's part is reduced, since anger arises when there is discrepancy between what you expect versus what you get. We are simply still dealing with the hand we've been dealt. It serves us well to think of special needs kids as "works in progress."

☐ *Overcome a fear of "coddling."* Parents and teachers are often afraid of doing harm by helping too much. How much help is appropriate? When does the role of caregiver end, and the role of the child take over? A mother of an ADHD child explained her confusion to me by way of the following question, "Am I supposed to harvest the food, grind it, chew it, *and* swallow it for her?"

Of course, children should be encouraged to accomplish everything that they can on their own. If they accomplish what they need to do, then we are done; if they do not, then we must step in, or make the first step smaller. Unfortunately, the "sink or swim" approach often does not work with kids in the syndrome mix. If they can't do it yet, then…they can't do it yet. We wouldn't tell a child with dyslexia, "We already went over phonics yesterday. Get it right today, or get an 'F.'" Similarly, negatively chastising a child with an autistic spectrum disorder for making the same social blunder as he made yesterday is not effective or useful. If it is a disability, it isn't going to be overcome tomorrow any more than will my own need for reading glasses.

Don't worry about making their life too easy. Even with our help, these kids will still be getting more than their fair share of practice of dealing with failures, frustration, criticism, and pain. We should only wish that our interventions for special needs kids could be so successful that their life will now be easier than everyone else's.

☐ ***Provide a safety net.*** The concept of a "safety net" may also help family/teachers overcome a fear of coddling. Let's try a few analogies. When acrobats are taught a new trapeze act, their trainers provide them with a safety net. Even Olympic gymnasts have a "spotter" when they perform their high bar routines. No one worries that providing these safeguards will interfere with learning, or will make the performer take her task less seriously. It is simply that without a safety net, the penalty for missing a handgrip while flying across the trapeze bars is neither commensurate with the mistake nor productive. Similarly, we may need to intervene in the child's college application process, because the penalty of messing up his future career is not commensurate with the "sin" of poor organization.

So, you should be the safety net or "spotter" for the special needs kid. If she gets it right, she won't need you, and there's no harm in you standing by. If she doesn't get it right, you are there to provide a softer landing—and make sure that the consequence is appropriate to the mistake. Let's take the example of a mother providing a safety net by nightly double-checking that her child correctly packed all of his homework for school. If the child has already packed away all of his work correctly on his own, then the mother has not interfered with any of the child's learning process; but, on the occasion that the student is actually missing an assignment, thank goodness she was there. There is a good outcome either way. Not a crutch, but a safety net. Knowing that there is a safety net and unconditional love will enable the child to actually take more risks.

☐ ***Teach "effective interdependence,"*** a term coined by Hallowell and Jensen (2008) to denote that no one is or should be totally independent. I'm a successful physician, but I rely on my family, secretaries, doctors, lawyers, and accountants, etc. We need to teach and model how children can ask for help when they need it, and how to offer back what they have to give in return. That's life. Let's learn it early. I should add that when your child grows up, you may need to be replaced by a secretary, girlfriend, or wife—hopefully not all at the same time!

☐ *Explain to the child that it's not his "fault," but it is still his "problem."* Being sure the child understands this may also help overcome the fear of coddling: he still owns the consequences of his problems; he just doesn't have to feel worthless because of them. Explain that, "Just because we're not angry and we understand why your brain works this way, it doesn't mean you don't suffer the problematic consequences." For example, it may not be an ADHDer's fault that he lost his homework (disorganization is part of ADHD), but he still has the problem of a lower grade or having to do it again.

☐ *Communication between teacher and parent is key.* In order to provide the appropriate safety net and teach effective interdependence, teachers and parents will need to communicate. Use phone calls, email, memo notebook, or anything else...but stay in touch! Waiting for mid-term progress reports is too late for the parents to help the child dig herself out of the problem. Don't expect the special needs child to be a reliable purveyor of information.

☐ *A teacher can make or break a child's year.* Don't *underestimate* your role in a child's success. I cannot tell you how many times parents and special needs students tell me, "Some years were great; others were unmitigated disasters." When I ask why, the answer is overwhelmingly, "In the successful years, he felt that his teacher really understood him and was rooting for him. In the disaster years, he didn't click with the teacher, and just completely shut down."

☐ *Don't necessarily overestimate your role in a child's failures.* Factors out of your control may be at play: there may be problems with academic, personal, or family stresses; or medications may not be working. Teachers, try your best, re-evaluate your strategy with parents and with the school's guidance departments, and then just keep plugging away.

Despite the best efforts of teachers, parents, and even the child, some problems cannot be totally fixed—at least not this year, anyway. Sometimes, there are just "least bad" strategies.

☐ *If it is working, keep doing it. If not, do something else.* This is hard work, but you will make it through this; you have no choice. Failure is not an option. However, don't expect that all problems can be fixed overnight. Many of these kids will be "works in progress" as part of a "50-year plan."

☐ *Forgive yourself.* Dr. Barkley urges his readers to forgive themselves nightly for their inability to be perfect (Barkley 2013, p.167). Each night, review how you've done that day and how you could do better. Then, remember that each of us is only human, and forgive yourself for the past. This applies to parents, children, and teachers. The child needs parents who feel good enough about themselves that they have enough energy left to positively and calmly help their offspring.

☐ *Review this book, and others, periodically.* You are going to forget this stuff, and different principles will likely be needed at different stages.

Understanding the child's mindset

☐ *Learn about the child's problems.* As you learn about the child's areas of difficulty, you will feel more confident in your teaching/parenting methods, and feel less threatened. Also, you will probably find that many of the difficult behaviors are actually part of the child's underlying diagnosis. For example, you might have "blamed" a child with Asperger's for taking on the role of "class policeman," until you discover that this black-and-white rigidity is a typical part of the syndrome.

This book is a great place to start learning. Further reading suggestions are given in Appendix 4. The school's special education staff should also have recommended materials for classroom teachers and parents.

☐ ***Seek to understand.*** Ask yourself, "Why did he do that?" There is *always* a reason, even if that reason is neither rational nor productive in the long term. For example, a child with dyslexia may act up whenever the reading becomes difficult. In the long term, that is a bad strategy, but in the short term, being sent to the principal solves the immediate discomfort of feeling inadequate. Often, the behaviors make sense if we remember that these children are so overwhelmed by what is happening right now that they live almost exclusively in the present, without much room left for foresight into future consequences.

☐ ***Remember that the child is most likely stressed out by his own behavior.*** True, a child's stress may have been brought upon himself, but it is still an unpleasant stress. For example, a child's own disorganization may have caused him to be late for the bus, but rushing out of the house is still an unpleasant experience for him as well as for the parent. That stress may be taken out on whoever is standing by—you.

☐ ***Not all brains see everything as the same.*** A special needs child may not experience the world exactly as we do. Their abilities and coping skills may not be even across the board. Much of the behavior will strike us as odd, or different, or even inexplicable. You're right. That's why the kids may have a diagnosable condition.

What *is* the child's brain seeing? Although by no means always accurate, we can open a window into a child's mind simply by carefully paying attention to—and legitimizing— his reaction. Unfortunately, we often incorrectly dismiss their reaction as irrelevant by labeling it "over-reacting."

People do not "over-react." Instead, they "over-feel." When a child blows up over what seems like a trivial issue to us, it may help us to understand that in *this* child's mind, this issue must have a tremendous amount of meaning. He's not acting. We could benefit from saying, "Wow, if that's how it feels to him, we should calmly discuss this!"

☐ *We see only part of what is going on in a child's life.* By the time a kid with issues arrives in class, who knows what has gone on already that morning or the previous evening at home? Waking up and getting dressed may have involved major fights. Homework may have comprised hours of frustration for everyone. And when the child comes home, the parent needs to remember that their special child may have had an especially difficult time at school. So, first we must seek to understand, and then we plan a reaction.

☐ *Ask yourself, "Would I want to be talked to the way I am talking to my child?"* Put yourself in your child's shoes. Ask yourself, especially if you were already overwhelmed, "Would I want anyone to treat me in the way I am treating my child?" (Brooks and Goldstein 2001, pp.18–19). Would you? Really? How would it make you feel?

☐ *Also, ask yourself, "Am I saying or doing things in a way that would make my children the most receptive to listening to what I have to say and learning from me?"* (Brooks and Goldstein 2001, pp.18–19). A negative or angry tone is unlikely to increase a child's acceptance of your instruction.

☐ *Finally, remember that some of the difficult child/adolescent behavior is simply normal.* We may be quick to assume all difficult moments with the child are due to some "disorder." Keep in mind, though, that life with any child is never totally smooth. Every family up and down the street, and every teacher up and down the hallway, is having some problems as well. That may be comforting; it's nice to know that you are not alone.

In particular, even typical pre-teens and teens go through a period when their respect for adult authority is less than maximal. Anecdotal experience suggests that, from the typical child's perspective:

» when the child is under ten years old, Mom/teacher seems to know *everything*

» when the child is around ten years old, Mom suddenly seems to know *less than nothing*

» when the child returns from college, *Mom* seems to have learned *a fair amount* while he was away, and seems to be a pretty good source of advice.

How to change the child's behavior

There are two major rules for affecting a child's behavior.

1. Keep it positive.

2. Keep it calm.

It sounds simple enough!

Rule 1: Keep it positive

☐ *Enjoy the child.* Seek to enjoy, not to be frustrated. Celebrate the child's humor, creativity, passion, and even her unique qualities. Given all of the child's problems, it is sometimes hard to find anything to praise. Find some accomplishment to sincerely laud, and some activity to enjoy together. You know, "Catch them being good." Laugh with each other. Let the youngster be helpful and "useful." Let the child know that you believe in him, despite the difficulties.

In her autobiography, Liane Holliday Willey explains: "The people who have proven that they will stand by me no matter what I say, think or do, have given me a finer gift than they will ever realize" (Willey 1999, p.58). This may not always be easy, but remember the saying of a retired teacher, "The children who need love the most will always ask for it in the most unloving ways" (Barkley 2013, p.5).

☐ *Remediate the strengths.* Many parents would not hesitate to drag their child to a tutor to work on a difficult academic skill—say biology—with the ultimate goal of improving a child's self-esteem. But if our goal is to provide our child/

student with successful life experiences and strengths, why work only on the skills that are hard for them? As stated by a youngster in a cartoon (www.livesinthebalance.org/sites/default/files/stickers.pdf), "Why do I only get stickers for doing things that I'm not good at?" Why not encourage at least as much those skills that come naturally to a child—even if they are not the ones we had dreamt for our child to have. Who knows? Maybe these "islands of competence," such as music or constructing things, could be the basis of a future career or friendships. After all, future employers don't chose employees by asking them what is their weakest skill, but rather what strengths can they bring to the job (Brooks and Goldstein 2001, pp.135–166). Similarly, friends are chosen on the basis of common interests, not on areas of disability. In any case, doesn't it make sense to spend resources on building success through natural skills, rather than solely hammering away at skills that come less naturally?

Brooks and Goldstein (2001) also point out that this applies to the schools as well. In many students' Individualized Education Plans (IEPs), there is a section listing a child's strengths and weaknesses. Many people think that listing the child's strengths is merely an attempt to soften the blow before the school tells the parents about the weaknesses or, alternatively, to list skills that don't need attention because they are already good. However, following Brooks and Goldstein's logic, shouldn't these strengths be celebrated, encouraged, and built upon by the school and others? For example, if a child is already an exceptional reader, then rather than ignore reading, wouldn't it make sense for the system to build even further upon the skill? After all, those are the skills that will ultimately make the world a better place. If nothing else, though, success in these islands of competence—be they athletic or academic—is likely to improve a child's attitude, and thus performance, in all areas.

☐ *Focus on "mirror traits."* Hallowell and Jensen (2008) suggest re-labeling negative traits with positive mirror traits. For example, he's not *distractible*, he's *curious*. Or, he's not *disorganized*, he's *spontaneous*. Or, he's not *intrusive*, he's *eager*. You get the idea.

☐ **Remember that their "disability" is also responsible for many of their strengths.** For example, autism spectrum disorder may account for a person's outstanding technical knowledge, and ADHD may be at the heart of a person's boundless energy. Conditions in the syndrome mix are a part of who a person is—both enviable as well as unenviable traits.

☐ *Use positive reinforcement when possible.* Instead of negatively reinforcing wrong behavior, Barkley reminds us to set a reward for the correct behavior you would rather replace it with (Barkley 2013, p.211). For example, suppose that you are trying to correct a child's nasty behavior towards his sister. Your goal is that he should be nice to her. So, rather than punishing the child for yelling at his sister, positively reward him for each kind comment. Rewards should be immediate, frequent, powerful, clearly defined, and consistent.

Younger children may respond to sticker charts or token systems. Greene's criteria for adopting behavior modification/reward systems are summarized below (1999).

» The behavior must be worth the effort of changing.

» The child must have the ability to consistently control the behavior.

» The reward/punishment is likely to work (e.g., punishment is unlikely to correct forgetful behavior).

» Those with allegedly cooler heads can apply the plan consistently.

» It is the child's problem.

When using reward/token systems, remember the following points:

» Most people are drawn towards the most attractive stimulus. Reward systems capitalize on this trait by using a "carrot" to lead the child in a productive direction.

» "But don't 'bribes' lead them to do things for the wrong reasons?" Yes, but they already haven't responded to the "right" reasons. That appeal has already failed by the time enticements are added.

» Children with special needs particularly require frequent, strong, and immediate feedback and rewards.

» The rules need to be succinctly reviewed at the scene before they are needed.

» The rewards will need frequent rotation to maintain their power.

» Enticements can be as simple as, "First we work, then we get to play." Or, "If you only tease your sister twice this week, then you get your allowance."

Formal systems are described in many books, including those by Dr. Russell Barkley (see Further Reading). Token systems entail earning points for good behavior (or losing them for bad behavior) that are then traded in for any privilege. Practically speaking, formal token systems are difficult to maintain, and work best with elementary school children. The school psychologist can help with specifics. Be careful, though: if sticker/reward systems do work, then people tend to stop using them, and the problem returns. Success is its own worst enemy.

☐ *Recognize that children already do well if they can.* Reward systems can fail because they mistakenly assume that a child's misbehavior is due to a lack of motivation, and thus that changing the reward (i.e., the motivator) will subsequently change the behavior—as if the rewards of getting praised by teachers and parents, getting As, getting into a good college, getting a good job, and getting a nice house with a pool aren't enough incentive already. A child's inability to sit through a lesson or to tolerate frustration is not likely to be due to a lack of adequate motivators. It is much more probable that the misbehavior comes from lacking a skill set—such as lacking the ability to attend or the skill to think flexibly. Children already do well if they can (Greene 2010). It is better to work on the underlying skill set that the child is having trouble with. See, well, the rest of this book for how to do that.

☐ *Negative reinforcement does not improve attitude.* Threats may change behavior, but they do not motivate towards a good attitude. Only the rewards of success (internal or external) lead to an improved mood. Do you want to see your child's/student's attitude and performance plummet? Try taking away their islands of success (such as sports or theater) as negative punishment.

☐ *Set realistic, achievable goals.* One downtrodden patient of mine perked up to say, "My parents do 'disappointment' really well." Avoid disappointment by setting realistic, achievable goals. This is part of accepting your child for who she is, not necessarily who you dreamt she would be. Yes, it would be nice if your child were better at academics or more tolerant, but isn't there enough good stuff left to celebrate anyway? Let her know.

☐ *Avoid the "resentment treadmill."* Resentment breeds resentment. Perhaps, the following sounds familiar.

> John is nasty to his mom. Mom stays quiet. John is nasty again. This time, Mom yells back. The next morning, Mom is still angry. She walks into the John's bedroom and says, "Why can't you even set your own alarm clock? After how you treated me yesterday, you still expect me to wake you up?" John is bewildered—after all, he hasn't even got out of bed yet and his mom is yelling at him. He curses at his mother. John goes to school, acts disrespectfully (again), and gets in trouble with the teacher, who is still sensitized from yesterday's unpleasant classroom interaction.

Good morning! It's another day on the resentment treadmill.

By the time someone is reading this chapter, the resentment treadmill may have been running at high speed for some time. Each "side" (child or caregivers) can recite a litany of truly legitimate complaints against the other. As a ten-year-old patient of mine with Asperger's commented about a peer he wasn't getting along with, "We're both on each other's problem list."

The cycle leads nowhere good. Everyone can agree on that. Someone has to get off the treadmill first. Guess who it isn't going to be: the dysfunctional child. That leaves the mature adult to take the first leap. That's you. Don't look around; there's no one else reading this page. Oh, and by the way, don't expect instant results or gratitude. So, when tempted to fight fire with fire, remember that the fire department usually uses water!

Below are some strategies to help resist the appeal of jumping back on the treadmill. It's all easier said than done: resentment and anger can be addictive.

» **Why do adults think that only the child should change?** The kids aren't always wrong. Their points of view on some issues may be more legitimate than ours. That may be hard for us to accept. After all, those people who *think* they are always right are annoying to those of us who *are* always right! Maybe *we* should teach flexibility by example.

» **Don't be a nasty cop** (Carver 2005). Imagine being pulled over by a policeman for making an illegal turn. The policeman approaches your window, hands you the ticket, and proceeds to insult you. "Don't you have any respect for the safety of yourself or others? Don't you care about anything? You are always such a jerk! And, your car looks really disgusting! Why don't you clean it up?" What would you think about the policeman? Would you want to have dinner with him tonight? Would you want to give him a hug at bedtime? Would you look forward to seeing him in school tomorrow? Moral of the story: as you hand out the punishment, skip the nasty attitude. The punishment is bad enough. The nasty attitude just breeds resentment.

» *Avoid Dr. Phelan's four cardinal sins* (Phelan 1994, p.39).

1. Don't nag. It hasn't worked yet. If you don't have anything nice to say, don't say it. Even simple comments like "How was your day?" may cause frustration in your child.

2. Don't lecture. It doesn't work either. Plus, given their sense of time, ADHDers will find the experience interminable. Instead, give one or two brief, clear instructions. "Insight transplants" from you to your child, as Phelan calls them, are unlikely to work.

3. Don't argue. It takes two to fight. No argument can take place without your consent.

4. Don't offer unscheduled, spontaneous "advice." What are the odds that your Nintendo-playing teen will respond pleasantly to your request to discuss, right now, that school project due next month?

Phelan calls these four points "The Four Cardinal Sins." These "sins" are ineffective, annoying, and thus actually harmful. Why would we use them? Instead, either decide that the issue is aggravating but not significant enough to warrant intervention (i.e., stay quiet); or make an appointment with your child to discuss the issue (see the upcoming collaborative problem-solving approach on page 49).

» *Minimize arguments with the "no-fault" approach.* Chris Zeigler Dendy (2006) has the very useful suggestion that rules be enforced with a no-fault approach. In other words, avoid arguments based on whose fault it is. Just deal with the end results. Consider this scene where a teen has a 10pm curfew, and he arrives home at 11:45pm.

Teen: "I'm sorry, Mom. I was getting a ride home from Jack, and he had to stop for gas. Jill had a stomachache and we had to drop her off at her house. Then, Jack remembered that he had to stop for milk for his baby brother. I couldn't call because my cell phone battery died. So, I'm sorry that I'm late."

How do you argue with that set of excuses? You can't. Instead, proceed as follows.

Mom: "I'm sorry, too. I'm sorry that you had bad luck. I'm sorry that you are stuck with the punishment we've agreed on if you come home past your curfew. I'm not blaming you, but those are the rules. Now, let's go have a snack."

It doesn't matter why a child arrives late. He is late, this is the consequence, and we'll try to create a plan to prevent it from happening again. It eliminates negative discussion, doesn't it?

This approach is particularly useful when dealing with people who blame others for their problems, as do many people with ADHD, for example. There is no point in *their* blaming *you* if blame is not being made relevant. Could this be unfair? Sometimes, yes. But in the long run, arguments are diminished, and that is to everyone's advantage.

This approach also prevents direct criticism of the child. We punish the end behavior and its end results but are not directly criticizing the child. After all, we are not assigning blame to anyone. Thus, this approach is a rediscovery of the old adage, "Criticize the behavior, not the child." It is another way to keep things positive.

» *Keep your relational bank account in the positive.* It may help to consider that you have a bank account of experiences with the child: there are good times and bad times that can be deposited into your relationship. Your goal is to have the overall balance in the positive. Make sure that you take the good times with the bad. When she is finally ready to apologize, talk, or cuddle, take her up on her offer right then and there. Your goal is to put some good times into your relationship. Take them as they come. Otherwise, you end up only with the bad.

As you enter into each interaction, ask yourself, "Will my next comment/action make my bank account with the child run into debt or into a positive flow? Am I about to jump back on the resentment treadmill?" If so, is it worth it?

» ***Provide help for deficits at the moment it is needed.*** Children with special difficulties need enabling at the time of need, not negative feedback when it is already too late. Unfortunately, the simple reality is that negative consequences do not usually teach kids with disabilities the behaviors they need. Typically, they *know* what to do; they just cannot carry out the plan. They already know, for example, that they should come to class prepared. They already know that if they do not do their homework, they will not get into the good college that they want. However, for them, it just does not happen. Punishing such a child would make as much sense as punishing a child with dyslexia for not remembering the difference between a "b" and a "d." (Note that in the US, federal law prohibits a school from punishing a child for symptoms of a disability.)

Once we understand that negative reinforcement has not been working, we are ready to provide relief for their disabilities by guiding them at the moment guidance is needed—rather than continued disbelief that they did it wrong again. We may be amazed at how many times the kids keep using the same unsuccessful strategies, but how many times is it going to take for *us* to figure out that *we* keep using unsuccessful strategies with them?

» *Punishment is not your chance to inflict misery; it is your chance to improve your child's upcoming decisions.* What is the purpose of punishment? Unless you are a sadist, you are not really trying to "get even" or to make little kids miserable. Rather, the purpose of a punishment presumably is to correct future behaviors. A modest, immediate punishment is likely to be at least as effective as a prolonged one. A spiral of increasing punishments is unlikely to work, and just saddles everyone with a lengthy period of unhappiness in the future. Consider the following scenario:

> Father: "If you don't apologize right now, there will be no TV tonight."
>
> Child gives no response.
>
> Father: "Okay. If you don't apologize in the next ten seconds, there will be no TV this entire week."
>
> Child gives no response. Soon, the punishment is up to no TV for a month. There is still no apology, the child has a meltdown, and everybody is angry.
>
> Twenty-nine days of no TV pass. The family has been miserable.
>
> Child: "Dad, do you remember what I'm being punished for?"
>
> Father: "Johnny, I don't have a clue."

The punishment has far exceeded its usefulness, don't you think? Remember, when punishment is required, keep it immediate and controlled.

Much more useful than punishment is to work on the underlying problem that set off the misbehavior. This work should not be attempted in the heat of the moment. We will need to invoke Rule 2: keep it calm.

45

Rule 2: Keep it calm

☐ **Be a defusing influence, not an inflammatory one.** The life of a special needs child is overwhelming. The treatment for his over-reaction is to defuse the situation, not inflame it. This applies whether the child has ADHD, autism spectrum disorder, oppositional defiant disorder, bipolar disorder, anxiety disorder, or just about any condition. Actually, this principle applies to just about any human interaction.

Seek to defuse, not to inflame. When tempers or anxieties flare, allow everyone to cool off—including the caregiver. By analogy, when the kitchen pot is about to boil over, you don't turn the heat up! Rather, you take the pot off of the stove until things safely settle down. Only then do you attempt to gently stir the pot.

Productive discussion can only occur during times of composure. You might think that stressing a child would force him to "give in" and reach the right decision, but experience and science prove otherwise. Arnsten (2005) showed in animals that slightly increasing dopamine levels in the brain, as occurs with mild stress, helped to improve the animals' "executive function." (See Chapter 3 on ADHD for more about executive functions.) However, pushing brain dopamine levels too far, such as would occur with excessive stress, actually lowers executive function. Thus, physiologically, excessive stress pushes mammals away from the same clear thinking that you are trying to help the child achieve. Don't do it! How clearly do you think when you are over-stressed? Do you make the best long-term decisions during the heat of the moment?

Remember: negative behaviors usually occur because the child is spinning out of control, not because he is evil. For kids that Dr. Ross Greene (2010) refers to as "explosive," the first step, then, is to "Just *stop!*" (Although most typical children will respond well to typical enticements and threats of punishment, if you made it this far, your child probably isn't one of them.) Here, our focus is on *preventing* overheated meltdowns. We anticipate problems and try to head them off: we stop, we stay calm, and we negotiate (if possible, well in advance, before the problems recur).

Here are some details of a defusing technique—based on "Plan B" by Dr. Ross Greene (2010).

☐ *Head off big fights before they begin.* When things start going badly, redirect to a positive direction rather than criticizing the misbehavior. For example, if the child is arguing with a peer, then suggest a new activity such as having a snack, rather than handing out a punishment.

☐ *Pick your fights.* Is this fight worth chipping away at your relationship with the child for? Remember, this is not war. Psychologist Dr. Steven Covey (1989) reminds parents to keep in mind what you want your child to think about you when he delivers your eulogy. If you are a teacher, keep in mind how you want the child to remember the school year.

☐ *Give transition warnings.* Many special kids have trouble with transitions. Discuss in advance what is expected. Give plenty of warnings. Have the child repeat out loud the terms he just agreed to. Some children need to negotiate for those "two more minutes." A little extra patience on the caregiver's part may help avoid a useless, more time-consuming meltdown. Consider a timer.

☐ *Watch the "stress speedometer."* Imagine that a child (or you) is a car with a stress speedometer. When that speedometer reaches 60 miles per hour (mph), the back wheels will spin out and nothing can prevent a crash. Attempts to intervene during the spin out will just prolong the system failure. The goal, then, is to keep anyone from hitting 60 mph. So imagine you enter the scene when the child is at a stress level of 40 mph. For the child, the anxiety of the current situation is getting to him. You laugh—or you divert, or you negotiate—and the stressometer comes down to 30 mph. Great! You are on the right track. Keep it up. However, the next day, the same intervention brings the child up to 50 mph. Back off! You are just a moment away from the 60 mph point of no return, and the horrible meltdown that will then be unstoppable. Just *stop*, and walk away.

This is not the time to give in to our impulse to just get done with it. You might have the self-control to do that, but your special child may not have been born that way. Don't assume that just because you can handle it, he can as well. All brains have equal rights, but all brains are not constructed in the same way.

☐ *"Just stop!" is the key—for the overwhelmed person and for you.* Incredible things happen if everyone is able to just stop:

» It works! Even five or ten minutes are all most people require to regain their composure and ability to think clearly. These few minutes spent to avoid a crisis certainly beat enduring a much more negative and lengthier meltdown.

» With the benefit of time, most people will come around to the right conclusion on their own, and comply.

Once you have calmed down, the correct method of behavioral management will seem almost blatantly obvious. For example, we try to keep it positive. We discuss seeking to understand and making the child part of the problem-solving process. We discuss choosing only productive punishments. When you are calm, these approaches are not exactly rocket science, and are almost self-evident.

"But what if he doesn't just stop?" Encourage compliance with the system by explaining in advance that this cooling off period is not a punishment. It is not like the old punitive "time out" in the corner system, which works best with preschool and elementary school-age students. Rather, the child gets to go and do some pleasant—yet soothing—activity. You may need your own soothing activity, too. The earlier you can disengage, the easier it will be. Warning symptoms that someone is becoming overloaded and needs a break are not particularly obscure. They usually contain subtle clues, such as, "Just stop! Leave me alone!" They're telling you what their brain needs right now in no uncertain terms. Exactly which of those words don't we adults understand?

After stopping, state the rule once and leave. The decision to declare a cooling off period has nothing to do with a decision as to who "won." You are not giving in. Come back later when cool heads prevail to teach the following amicable problem-solving technique to your child.

Ross Greene's collaborative problem-solving technique

Congratulations! Everyone has stopped. Once everyone's dopamine levels have been allowed to return to normal, you may find that everyone is in agreement and is complying. If not, here are some details on Greene's three-step negotiating technique (2010), to be attempted only in moments of calmness. This is where the real teaching occurs.

1. *Invite the child to state his problem, and then the adult should acknowledge the concern.* Some children may need help in formulating their issue, especially those on the autism spectrum. However, having the child state what's bothering her is only half of step one. The other half is for the adult to express empathy for that problem—not necessarily capitulating that the child is right—just that her feelings and needs are recognized. A simple recitation of what the child said, or an, "I hear you," may suffice, but a better way to show that you are really seeking to understand is to keep "drilling" for helpful information. Show that you are trying to put yourself in their shoes and understand exactly what is bothering them.

2. *The parent puts his view on the table.* Similarly, the child does not have to agree, rather just recognize her parent's point of view that will have to be dealt with.

3. *The child is invited to come up with multiple possible, doable, win-win solutions to solve any mismatch between the child's and the adult's view of the problem.* He should then evaluate each and bounce his ideas off of the adult. Don't worry about losing control: the adult always gets to concur with which compromise is accepted.

In doing this, caregivers will be modeling negotiation, not inflexibility. What is wrong with teaching a child to be flexible and to seek win-win solutions? The goal is for the child to internalize the above process.

This collaborative approach to problem solving can also be used to address specific lagging skill sets. For example, a mother might notice that her child with autism spectrum disorder doesn't have sufficient skill at making friends. She might approach the child by asking, "I've noticed that you haven't had many playdates recently. What's up?" The child is thereby invited to state his problem (step one), "I don't like playdates because the other kids play with each other and ignore me." In step two, the mother responds, "My concern is that avoiding playdates will only make it harder for you to learn how to make friends." For step three, the mother could invite the child to throw out possible solutions to the problem. Eventually, he might come up with solutions such as only have one child over at a time, or have the sibling who always interrupts be out of the house, etc. Thus the collaborative problem-solving process can be used to address either specific problems as they arise (such as fighting with a sibling) or to address underlying, problematic skill sets.

Some research (Brown 2009, p.75) shows the best results with the fewest "dropouts" from treatment are achieved by combining the collaborative problem-solving approach with behavior management training—the latter including:

- educating parents on the true nature of ADHD or other problems

- setting up the difference between non-negotiable behaviors (drugs, alcohol, violence, respect, etc.) versus those behaviors that can be negotiated

- parents and child spending time together without being critical—to break the negative cycle of interactions

- "catching the child being good"

- reward systems preferentially rewarding positive behaviors, etc.

Using Plan B in the classroom

Hopefully, these techniques will not be required too often in class. Using them proactively in private will tend to head off problems (after all, they're usually predictable) before bursting out again in front of peers. We are only talking about the rare classroom situation where there is simply not much of an alternative. Certainly, it is difficult to let one student appear to "get away with it" in front of other students. However, having the students witness an unproductive meltdown does not model a useful interaction, either. If the event is already "public," the adult should make it clear to everyone witnessing the situation that no one is "getting away" with anything. There will be discussion and consequences meted out, even though the discussion will take place later in private. We are modeling peaceful, useful, human interactions.

Quick quiz on angry behavior

This good-natured open book quiz is designed to test and reinforce your understanding of angry behavior. The questions relate to the following *true* story.

> A 13-year-old boy with ADHD discovers that his orthodontic bite-plate is missing from its handy container. He angrily accuses everyone else of having taken it. His mother explains the blatantly obvious fact that no one else would be interested in his used dental appliance. He continues screaming and blaming her for its absence.

1. Which of the following answers best explains the accusatory behavior of this otherwise bright child?

   a. He's not quite smart enough to comprehend that his bite-plate isn't worth stealing.

   b. He's overwhelmed by frustration.

2. Yelling back and accusing your child of behaving horribly would:

   a. cause him to say, "Oh, thanks for helping me see the error of my ways"

   b. cause him to be even more overwhelmed.

3. You try unsuccessfully to help find the bite-plate. A *useful* parental response at this point would be:

   a. engage in an escalating screaming match

   b. *stop*! Walk away. Retain your composure. Resist the urge to get the last word in. Resume discussion when everyone is calm.

4. This type of outrageous, explosive behavior in ADHD is the result of:

   a. a nasty, selfish child

   b. a common reaction of overwhelmed children.

5. Your goal as caregiver is to:

   a. further inflame the child's frustration, leading to a spiraling downhill relationship

   b. see yourself as a therapist, teaching the child to *stop* and defuse the situation.

6. In the heat of real life, would you have acted the correct way?

   a. Usually yes.

   b. Usually no.

Answers to all questions: b.

CHAPTER 3

Attention Deficit Hyperactivity Disorder

"Okay, Bobby has ADHD (attention deficit hyperactivity disorder). That explains why he doesn't seem to pay attention and is so fidgety. But I still don't understand so many things about him. Why is he so disorganized? Why won't he write down his homework assignments? Why doesn't punishing him seem to have any effect? Why doesn't he see the consequence of his actions? Why does his mother say that homework is such a fight? Is it true that he blows up so easily at home?"

Bobby's mom has ADHD, also. Once, while joking about her chaotic life, she said, "I aspire to have obsessive compulsive disorder—so that I might be more organized." She was serious.

Defining ADHD
"Official" (and woefully incomplete) definition of ADHD

The American Psychiatric Association gives "official" criteria for many syndromes in the *Diagnostic and Statistical Manual of Mental Disorders-5* (APA 2013), commonly referred to as DSM-5. As typically defined by DSM-5, ADHD consists of a triad of inattention and/or hyperactivity-impulsivity.

Symptoms of the "inattentive" type

- *Attention and distractibility problems are a core symptom of ADHD.* There is an inability to inhibit distractions in order to stay focused on the task at hand. The person does not seem to listen or pay close attention. There may be frequent careless mistakes.

- *Organizational difficulties are an equal part of the problem.* This includes difficulty organizing, sustaining, or completing tasks. The person may be forgetful, "absentminded," or easily lose things.

Symptoms of the hyperactive–impulsive type

- *Hyperactivity difficulties* include being fidgety or talking excessively. The child may run, climb, seem "on the go," or be out of the seat excessively. Additionally, he may have difficulty playing quietly. This may manifest in adults with ADHD as an internal sense of restlessness.

- *Impulsivity difficulties* include blurting out answers, difficulty waiting for turns, intruding, or interrupting.

In addition, at least several symptoms should begin before the child is 12 years old (DSM-IV used a cut-off of seven years old), interfere with overall life functioning, and occur in at least two settings (such as home, school, sports, etc.). DSM-5 also includes more adult type examples, such as noting that the criterion descriptive for children as "runs about or climbs" may instead present with the more typical adolescent/adult symptom of "feeling restless."

Using these criteria, DSM-5 defines three typical subtypes of ADHD, which are:

- ADHD, predominantly inattentive presentation

- ADHD, predominantly hyperactive/impulsive presentation (rare form)

- ADHD, combined presentation (both inattentive and hyperactive/impulsive—the most common form).

By current terminology, even if the person does not have hyperactivity, the diagnosis will still be "ADHD." The term "ADD" is no longer an official DSM term. DSM-5 now also adds the optional "specifiers" of mild, moderate, or severe, or in partial remission.

Note that *disorganization* is actually built into the definition of ADHD. In fact, it is fair to say that you really can't have ADHD unless you are disorganized or have to work especially hard at becoming organized. (I have found an exception to this rule may occur when an anxiety disorder about the future compensates for the ADHD inability to pay attention to anything except what is most fascinating right now.)

A more useful definition of ADHD

A problem with inhibition

Children with ADHD typically can pay attention to their video-games (or Lego®) forever. As long as they are allowed to stay at the most fascinating activity, they are fine. The problem, though, occurs when they are supposed to pay attention to something that is less captivating (e.g., multiplication), while simultaneously filtering out something that is more intriguing (e.g., the birds outside the window). That requires putting brakes on the "distractions."

Observations such as this have led Dr. Russell Barkley and others to define ADHD as a deficiency of *inhibition*, not a deficiency of attention span, per se (Barkley 1998, 2013). Kids (and adults) with ADHD, then, are relatively brakeless. They are:

- unable to put brakes on distractions → inattentive

- unable to put brakes on inside thoughts → impulsive

- unable to put brakes on *acting* upon distractions or thoughts → hyperactive.

These brakes reside in our brain's frontal and prefrontal lobes—the part of our brain just behind our forehead. These inhibitory centers keep us from being flooded by sensory information. They also allow us the luxury of time during which we can consider our options before reacting. Thus, unlike most other complex organisms, humans have the option of modulating their responses. In ADHD, though, the frontal and prefrontal lobes are essentially under-functioning. The inhibitory centers are asleep on the job. This is why one of my books is entitled *ADHD—Living without Brakes* (Kutscher 2009).

Therefore, the concept of ADHD as poor inhibition explains the classic symptoms of ADHD above, but also leads us to understanding the serious problems with other "executive functions" typically seen in ADHD.

Problems with "executive function"

What are "executive functions"? Our brain's frontal and prefrontal lobes function largely as our own Chief Executive Officer—as our own self-regulator. These frontal centers consider where we came from, figure out where we want to go, and plan how to control ourselves in order to get there. In short, executive functions are the skills we require to make a plan and actually execute it. They are the actions we direct at ourselves in order to alter our future for the better (Barkley 2013, p.56). Executive functions include the following self-regulatory skills (Barkley 2013; Brown 2009; Kutscher 2009).

- *The ability to inhibit*—the ability to put brakes on our behavior, is a skill of great importance in its own right. This inability to inhibit leads to the classic symptoms of ADHD that we just discussed. *Of extreme additional importance, though, is that without the ability to inhibit, you also never get to stop long enough to exercise any of the other executive functions below. Thus, deficiency of inhibition will likely lead to a deficiency of these other executive functions.*

- *Foresight*—perhaps the quintessential executive function. It refers to the ability to predict one's future needs, and to predict the consequences of one's actions. Lack of foresight is a key part of ADHD problems. There is no such thing as "the past" or "the future"; there is only right now. In fact, Barkley's full definition of ADHD has been the inability to inhibit the present "with an eye to the future" (Barkley 2013, p.25). It's not that ADHDers do not care about the future. It's that, right now, the future does not exist.

- *Hindsight*—our ability to keep the success rates of previous strategies in our working memory. Without hindsight, we are doomed to keep making the same errors. Although everyone has the right to make the same mistake again, ADHDers may be accused of abusing the privilege.

- *Self-talk*—the ability to talk to ourselves. It is a mechanism by which we work through our choices using words. Toddlers can be heard using self-talk out loud. Eventually, this self-directed ability becomes internalized and automatic. However, ADHDers have not inhibited their reactions long enough for this skill to fully develop. Frequently, they are not making conscious logical choices—they are just reacting.

- *Working memory*—the myriad of things that our brain can juggle at any given moment. We need to juggle what is happening now, foresight, hindsight, etc. It is analogous to the four gigabytes of RAM (random access memory) on our computers (versus "long-term memory," which corresponds to our computer's much larger 500 gigabyte hard drive).

- *Prospective memory*—a relatively newly formed term for the ability to "remember to remember." For example, we plan (or "intend") to pick up milk on the way home tomorrow, but we have to remember to actually do it. It's the brain's alarm clock.

- *Problem solving*—without the skills of hindsight, foresight, self-talk, and working memory to hold it all together, ADHDers have trouble with the process of problem solving, which is: state the problem, list your options, chose an option, carry out the plan, and evaluate/ reward yourself regarding your effort.

- *Organization (planning)*—problems are virtually guaranteed in ADHD. In fact, looking at the diagnostic criteria, it is nearly impossible to have ADHD without an element of disorganization. It starts to become more evident in late elementary school, and even more so in middle school. In middle school, the child's single elementary teacher (a.k.a. surrogate mother from 8am to 3pm) gets replaced by a team of teachers. Just at this time of need for increased amounts of organizational support, most schools pull back—adopting the "he needs to sink or swim on his own" attitude. (Unfortunately, kids with the disability we call ADHD will usually keep sinking without organizational support.)

- *Sense of time*—extremely poor in ADHD. Time can drag on f-o-r-e-v-e-r, or it can go by too quickly. Not all of us experience time in the same fashion.

- *Persistence*—the ability to stick with a project until completion.

- *Shifting from agenda A to agenda B*—a difficult task requiring good executive function. Pulling yourself out of one activity and switching to another—transitioning—is innately difficult, and requires effort and control.

- *Separating emotion from fact*—every fact or event has an *objective* significance, and also a *subjective emotional* significance that our brain tags it with. For example, a traffic jam has an objective reality of a 20-minute time delay. Different minds, though, give different emotional tags to the event. Some see the traffic jam as a nice way to relax a little more, whereas others see it as one more intentional act of cruelty imposed personally upon them by the universe. Without the gift of time, we never get to separate emotion from fact, and self-direct our emotional reaction. This leads to poor ability to judge the significance of what is happening to us.

- *Adding emotion to fact*—emotions motivate us to action, and difficulty with internalizing emotions makes it harder to motivate oneself and demonstrate ambition. Put another way, Brown (2009) describes the executive function difficulties in ADHD to include trouble with self-regulation *of* and *by* emotion.

Real-life symptoms of ADHD and executive dysfunction

We have just given the definitions of executive functions, but let's see how they play out in real life. As we show here, these problems with executive function are not just "incidental" symptoms. They are hard to live with—ask the teacher, parent, or child—and they are all commonly seen as part of the condition we summarize as "ADHD."

- *Lack of foresight*—"Bobby, you'll never get into a good college if you all you do is stare out of the window. Can't you see that you'd better start working on your term paper already? And why didn't you tell me that you need report covers for tomorrow? You act like your own worst enemy!" Foresight is a major adaptive ability of humans. Lack of use of this ability can be the most devastating part of ADHD. Teachers and mothers—often endowed with great foresight—are crushed as they watch the child repeatedly head down counterproductive paths. ADHD children are usually extremely poor at anticipating their needs!

- *Failing to remember future events*—"Bobby, the only thing I asked you to do all week was pick up the clothes from the cleaners on Wednesday, and you couldn't even be bothered to remember to do that."

- *Burn bridges in front of them*—"Bobby, you yell at me all day and now you expect me to drive you to karate?" Lots of typical people burn their bridges behind them. That's not a good idea, but unfortunately it is common. It takes executive dysfunction, though, to burn your bridges before you even realize that you are going to need them.

- *Poor hindsight/trouble learning from mistakes*—"Bobby, how many times do you have to be punished for the same thing? No matter how many times I give you a '0,' it doesn't ever seem to change your behavior." Unable to inhibit the present, Bobby cannot stop to consider lessons from the past.

- *Live at the "mercy of the moment"*—"Bobby is always swept away by whatever is happening to him right then and there. He's like a moth—smack up against the brightest light." ADHD behaviors make sense once we realize that they are based on reactions taking only the present moment into account. It is not that Bobby doesn't *care* about the future; it is that the future and the past don't even exist. Such is the nature of the disability.

  If you want to understand the ADHDer's actions, simply ask yourself: "What behavior makes sense if you feel as if you only have four seconds left to live?" By way of analogy, imagine happily fishing as you ride down a river. You would be so involved that you would not see the upcoming cliff. It's not that you don't "care" about falling over a cliff—it's that you don't even get to consider it. The future does not show up on your radar screen. Take the example in Figure 3.1.

This is what Jack sees: This is what everyone else seems to notice:

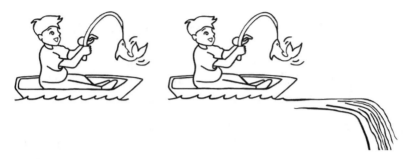

Figure 3.1 *The person with ADHD is so consumed by the present that he can't see the future coming up*

- *Poor organization*—"Bobby, don't you remember that there is a paper due tomorrow?!" And, "Why don't you come to me after class so that I can sign your assignment book?" And, "Why didn't you hand in your homework, even though your mother called me to say that you really did do it? Don't you care?"

- *Trouble finishing tasks*—"My husband starts a million projects but never finishes them." An ADHD mother stated that her nickname was "75%," because that's as far as any of her projects get.

- *Poor sense of time*—"Bobby, what have you been doing all afternoon? You can't spend two hours on the first assignment! You'll never make it to baseball practice!"

- *Time moves too slowly*—"This lecture is going on forever!"

- *Poor ability to utilize "self-talk" to work through a problem*—"Bobby, what were you thinking?! Did you ever think this through?"

- *Poor sense of self-awareness*—Bobby's true answer to the above question is probably, "I don't have a clue. I guess I wasn't actually thinking."

- *Poor reading of social clues*—"Bobby, you're such a social klutz. Can't you see that the other children think that's weird?"

- *Poor internalization and generalization of rules*—"Bobby, why do I need to keep reminding you that internet time comes *after* you finish your homework? And you'd think that, when I told you to clean out your desk, you would have known to clean out your cubby as well."

- *Inconsistent work and behavior*—"Bobby, if you could do it well yesterday, why is today so horrible?" With 100% of their energy, they may be able to control the task that most of us can do with 50% of our focus. But who can continually muster 100% effort? As the joke goes: ADHD children do something right twice, and we hold it against them for the rest of their lives (Barkley 2013, p.51).

- *Trouble with transitions*—"Bobby, why do you curse at me when I'm just calling you for dinner?"

- *Hyper-focused at times*—"When Bobby is on the computer, I can't get him off."

- *Poor frustration tolerance*—"Bobby, why can't you even let me help you get over this?"

- *Frequently overwhelmed*—"Please, just stop! I can't stand it. Just stop. Please!" In order to really feel what it must be like to be flooded by everything all at once, listen to the soundtrack that simulates the experience of ADHD at www.pediatricneurology.com/sound.htm. Then take the related survey with your child. It is a mind-altering experience that you cannot just read about.

Some real-life symptoms become more prominent in the older child (and at home).

- *Gets angry frequently and quickly*—"Bobby, why do you get so upset with your friends? Does it really have to be just your way?"

- *Pushes away those whose help they need the most*—"Mommy, stop checking my assignment pad. Get out!"

- *"Hyper-responsiveness"*—"Mommy, you know I hate sprinkles on my donuts! You never do anything for me! I hate you!" Barkley (2013) uses the term "hyper-responsiveness" to indicate that people with ADHD have excessive emotions. Their responses, however, are appropriate to what they are actually feeling. So next time you see someone "over-reacting," realize that they are actually "over-feeling," and must feel really awful at that moment.

- *Inflexible/explosive reactions*—"Bobby, you're stuck on this. No, I can't just leave you alone. Bobby, now you're incoherent. Bobby, just stay away. I can't stand it when you break things!" Greene (2010) gives an extensive explanation about the inflexible/explosive child.

- *Feels calm only when in motion*—"He always seems happiest when he is busy. Is that why he stays at work so late?"

- *Thrill-seeking behavior*—"He seems to crave stimulation at any cost. In fact, he feels most 'on top of his game' during an emergency."

- *Trouble paying attention to others*—"My husband never listens when I talk to him. He just cannot tolerate sitting around with me and the kids. He doesn't 'pay attention' to his family any more than he 'paid attention' in school." As the patient gets older, people in his life will increasingly expect more time and empathy to be directed their way. Yet, the above behaviors may interfere with the ADHDer's demonstration of these traits, despite his passions.

- *Trouble with mutual exchange of favors with friends*—without establishing a reliable "bank account" of kept promises, friendships can be hard to make.

- *Sense of failure to achieve goals*—"Somehow, I never accomplished all that I thought I could or should have." This deep disappointment is commonly what prompts adults with ADHD to seek help.

- *Lying, cursing, stealing, and blaming others*—these can become frequent accompanying problems for ADHDers; especially as the child gets older. Some particularly depressing data show how ADHD children compare with typical children. According to Barkley *et al.* (1990), 72% of kids with ADHD argue with adults (versus 21% of typical children); 66% of kids with ADHD blame others for their own mistakes (versus 17% of typical children); 71% of kids with ADHD act touchy or are easily annoyed (versus 20% of typical children); 40% of kids with ADHD swear (versus 6% of typical children); 49% of kids with ADHD lie (versus 5% of typical children) and 50% of kids with ADHD steal (versus 7% of typical children).

See Appendix 2 for a quiz designed to re-enforce your understanding about executive function's effect on school organization.

The rest of the iceberg: coping with family problems and co-morbidities

An ADHD child not only has the triad of inattention, hyperactivity, and impulsivity, but also must deal with other executive functions. As if that weren't enough, ADHD can be associated with any combination of the other conditions of the syndrome mix found in this book. As we have already seen, two-thirds of children with ADHD have at least one of these other "co-morbidities," and one-third of children with ADHD have at least two of them (Larson *et al.* 2011). Specifically, here's the likelihood of a child with ADHD also having:

- learning disabilities: 46%

- conduct disorder: 27%

- anxiety: 18%

- depression: 14%

- autism spectrum: 6%

- Tourette's syndrome: 1.3%.

(Larson *et al.* 2011)

Particularly commonly associated learning problems include the following:

- *Problems following a sequence of directions.* Consider the following typical directive from a teacher, "Okay, class. Be quiet, go to your seat, open your math book, turn to page 41, and do the first problem on the top of the page." The next thing you know, this kid is doing poorly in math because he is having trouble following a sequence of commands.

- *Poor handwriting.* Interestingly, this often improves with medication.

Even further, though, the child often has to deal with stressed-out parents who may have their own elements of the syndrome mix, and who are thus less than ideally prepared to meet the needs of their ADHD child. Interestingly, a recent study showed that medicating the ADHD *parent* improves the behavior of their ADHD *child* (New Clinical Drug Evaluation Unit 2013)! Besides their genes, the parent may additionally be stressed by trying to care for difficult family members. The last thing that a stressed-out child needs, though, is a stressed-out parent. Even if the child caused the parent's stress in the first place, it is one more problem that the child has to deal with.

The full ADHD picture, then, consists of classically defined ADHD, other executive functions including organization, co-morbidities, and family problems. If the only issues you are discussing with your doctor are hyperactivity and inattention, then the system is barely scratching the surface of the issues. No wonder that inattention has been considered to be just the tip of the ADHD iceberg (Kutscher 2009).

The "good" news comes from understanding that all of these problems are commonly part of the syndrome we call ADHD. They are nobody's fault—not yours, and not your child's. This understanding points the way towards coping with these issues.

Neurological basis of ADHD

No matter what country we look at, ADHD by DSM-IV criteria occurs in some 1 in 16 people (about 6%) (Barkley 2013, p.20). It is not just an American condition. Some specific prevalences are (Lecendreux 2011):

- US: 5–8% of children; 4–5% of adults
- France: 3.5–5.6%
- Finland: 6.6%
- Italy: 3.9%
- Spain: 14.4%.

Why does ADHD seem even more prevalent than that? Well, when one person in the home has ADHD, the whole family feels its effects. Assuming four people per family, that means that in any given home, there is a 4 in 16 risk that the household will be affected by someone with ADHD. That is how it works out: a condition that affects 6% of the population means that if four mothers get together, the odds are that one of their lives will be affected by ADHD in their family. That is a lot of families. Note that although 6% of the population has ADHD, only about 3% of the US school-age population is taking stimulant medication for the condition (Olfson *et al.* 2003).

As we have seen, ADHD results from insufficient functioning of the frontal and prefrontal lobes, and the other parts of the brain to which they connect, especially with the:

- basal ganglia (which help the brain to "coolly" sort out incoming information to deduce and hold in mind what is happening)

- limbic system (which determines the emotional reactions)

- cerebellum (which, amongst other things, controls the sense of time).

It appears that the frontal lobes have not been fully woken up by the neurotransmitters dopamine and norepinephrine. In turn, the frontal lobe brakes do not adequately inhibit other brain activity, thereby denying the brain of the ability for adequate self-directed regulation.

Interestingly, many of these same brain parts are involved in bladder control. Children with ADHD are almost three times as likely as non-ADHD children to have nocturnal bed-wetting (Shreeram 2009). Conversely, 40% of bed-wetters have ADHD (Baeyens 2004). Thus, children with ADHD should be evaluated for bed-wetting and vice versa.

It is well established that ADHD stems from a neurological basis. Adoption and other studies show a strong genetic component. If one member of the family has ADHD, each other first-degree relative (parent, sibling, or child) has roughly a 25% chance of having ADHD. Overall, genetics control about 80% of a person's risk for ADHD (Barkley 2013, pp.83–84). One possible contributor (it is unlikely that a single gene controls for ADHD) is a gene for the D4 dopamine receptor. PET (positron emission tomography) scans, blood flow studies, EEGs, MRIs and functional MRI scans all show prefrontal abnormalities.

Although these studies are not helpful in diagnosing an individual child, they should help us to be more understanding of the ADHDer's medically legitimate innate problems. It may come as a relief to parents that parenting skills have little to do with the *etiology* of ADHD, although parenting skills may have a lot to do with the *outcome*.

Treatment of ADHD and disorganization

Read Chapter 2, all of which applies to ADHDers. Plan B will be of particular importance to parents. Go ahead and read it again. Really. We'll wait. Often, parents and/or children may benefit from formal training programs such as cognitive behavioral therapy (CBT). In fact, parent training is typically the preferred initial treatment for preschool children (Charach 2013).

Presenting material to ADHD children

☐ *Clear the area of distractions.*

☐ *Present the material in a vibrant, animated, and attention-grabbing manner.* ADHD kids will attend to whatever is most stimulating to them at that moment. The adult's job is to make the information more interesting than, say, the paperclip on the table. (Have you ever noticed all of the fascinating shapes you can make by unraveling a paperclip?)

☐ *Allow preferential seating.* This is typically near the teacher, who is not always at the physical front of the classroom. For some children, though, being near the teacher means being near an overwhelming center of commotion. The preferred placement needs to be individualized, sometimes in direct discussion with the child. In general, modular seating with multiple students facing each other provides too much opportunity for distraction for ADHD children.

☐ *Establish good eye contact.* When asked, however, some children will be aware that eye contact actually interferes with their concentration. See what works best.

☐ *Tap on the desk* (or use another code) to bring the child back into focus.

☐ *Alert the child's attention with directives* such as, "This is important!"

☐ *Break down longer directions into simpler chunks.*

☐ *Check for comprehension.*

☐ *Encourage students to underline the key words of directions.*

☐ *Encourage students to mark incorrect multiple-choice answers with an "x" first.* This allows them to "get started" quickly, while forcing them to read all of the choices before making a final selection.

☐ *Allow physically hyperactive children out of their seats* to hand out and pick up papers, etc.

☐ *Allow for aerobic exercise.* Although ADHD does not stem from excess energy that needs to be worked off, research shows that vigorous exercise helps all children have better attention, including those with ADHD (Pontifex 2012).

Helping with organization

☐ *Recognize that disorganization is a major disability for almost everyone with ADHD.* In fact, the diagnostic criteria show that it is difficult to diagnose ADHD in the absence of organizational problems. Yes, ADHD students can—and frequently do—write a wonderful paper and then forget to hand it in. This striking unevenness in skills is what makes it a disability.

Keep plugging away at teaching organizational techniques that require *writing it down* somewhere rather than relying on the child's inconsistent memory. When the assignment pad isn't readily available, some kids manage to keep a piece of paper to scribble something on—and hopefully not lose it. A pad of Post-it® notes may work. For most students, though, a good organization system begins with the notebooks and assignment pads. If it's not written down, it doesn't exist.

School supplies

Too many notebooks are confusing and too heavy. I have never met a parent who doesn't complain (when asked) about the use of so many notebooks. ADHD students should have the following:

☐ *One notebook.* A single three-ring binder for all classes, with a divider between each subject. Ideally, no other binders! The student needs to date each sheet of paper as soon as he first touches it.

☐ *One bi-fold homework folder for all subjects* (one side marked clearly for all papers coming home, the other for all papers to be handed in). Unless there is one central location for paperwork to be brought home (or handed in), the ADHD child and his caregivers will never find it all.

☐ *An assignment book.* Make sure that they *use* it. See below.

☐ *A monthly calendar*, which can be filled in by the whole school team, or just downloaded blank from the school website or www.timeanddate.com. Each monthly calendar must be provided well in advance of the first of the next month. In fact, all students could benefit from training and supervision in the use of a monthly calendar for longer-range projects. On the monthly calendar, indicate dates to break larger projects into smaller sections (such as finish the reading, writing the rough draft, editing, etc.). Time is a very intangible concept—especially for ADHD children. Using a visual calendar helps make time more concrete, and allows the child to see upcoming deadlines, especially as they bunch up.

Assignments

Each day, the child and parent (and/or skills teacher) should look over the daily assignment pad as well as the monthly calendar of upcoming commitments and assignments. Any scraps of paper with notes on them should be rounded up and added to the list.

Next, convert the daily and monthly assignments into a time schedule for today. Look over the planner—including upcoming weeks—and write out the times that the child is going to actually accomplish tasks today. This provides a reality check for what can and cannot be crammed into one day. Note that what the child is planning to actually accomplish today may not correlate exactly with what is on today's assignment pad—some of the work that was assigned today doesn't need to be done today; but even more importantly, some of what has to be done today was assigned in the past.

☐ *Include time for eating, bathing, social websites, TV, etc.*

☐ *Factor in time for unexpected delays*—work taking too long, demands from parents, phone calls from friends, traffic jams, etc. The unexpected is expected.

☐ *Adhere to the time schedule.* This will help prevent taking diversions, since there is always an immediate deadline to meet.

☐ *The caregiver and child should go over this time schedule as soon as the child makes it* (which should be when coming home from school or in resource class). Children with ADHD typically have poor estimates of how long events will take. They will need our advice. Making this time schedule will allow them to see how well the estimates work out.

☐ *If the child is having trouble getting started* when she attempts to carry out the plan, then the first step is too big. Break the work down into smaller chunks, especially the early steps.

Until the child's organizational skills fully kick in—which is likely to take just a few more decades—the teacher and parent will need to "lend" their own frontal lobes to the child. This involves both *teaching* the skill to use assignment pads, and *supervising* it. The day that the caregivers stop supervising the creation of this time map is likely to be the day it stops being done. Remember the concept of executive function.

Assignment pads are not helpful if they are not filled out correctly. Ensure that parents and the child all know the correct assignment. Most students can take this responsibility upon themselves. Those with ADHD, though, usually cannot do it consistently. It is unfair and counterproductive to let intelligent students flounder because of this disability. Ask yourself, "Is the goal of this assignment to grade the kids on their ability to do physics and algebra; or are they being graded on their ability in an area of disability—to be self-organized?" Don't worry: the child is still responsible for getting it done. (When the ADHD children become adults, the wise ones will avail themselves of similar help from girlfriends, spouses, and secretaries—hopefully not all at the same time!)

The following options can be used to keep the child (and parent) informed of the assignments. This part will take effort, especially to keep the system going.

☐ *Inform the child about typical routines* (such as quizzes every Friday).

☐ *Hand out written assignments for the week.*

☐ *Put homework on the internet or school website.* That's not teaching the child to be overly dependent; it's what the professors usually do in college.

☐ *Initial students' homework assignment pads after each period.* Please do not expect the students to come up after class for the signature on their own. If they were organized enough to do that, we would not need to provide this accommodation. And, yes, the typical student is organized enough to come to the teacher, but this is not the typical student.

☐ *Practical experience shows that it is difficult to sustain a system of signing the homework pad.* If unable to initial all new assignments, then be sure to use the other systems above, and to address any occasionally missed work as below.

☐ *Notify the family immediately of any late assignments. This is key!* Waiting for a mid-term progress report is too late to correct the problem, and too late for the student to behaviorally notice the connection between his performance and the consequences. Use any of the following forms of communication.

» A phone call or email takes the child out of the loop, and works best. Email is particularly useful because teachers are hard to reach during the day, and a brief email note is certainly quicker than multiple missed phone call messages followed by an extended phone conversation.

» The parent could call the team leader/guidance counselor each week for an update.

» A "Comment Book" can be transferred back and forth daily for comments between the teacher and parent.

☐ *Allow for expedient makeup of late homework.* If deduction for lateness actually works to correct the problem, then keep doing it. If not, recognize the problem as a disability that is currently unable to be completely corrected. In such a case, the work does need to be completed, but is not fair for a persistent organizational disability to cause excessive and demoralizing deductions. Use one of two methods.

» Late work is accepted one day from direct parental notification.

» A non-punitive school detention can be assigned during which the work is done, and then accepted.

With either method, the student does all of the work (i.e., "gets away" with nothing), learns the material, and gets good grades. Without this support, the child "gets away" with not doing the work, does not learn the material, and gets bad grades. Isn't the more productive choice clear?

If, for some reason, it is necessary to give a failing grade for incomplete work, remember that 65% is failing, not 0%. Trying to get a decent quarterly grade while averaging in a "0%" or two is virtually impossible. For example, if a student gets four grades of 90% and just one 0%, her new average is 72%. Very demoralizing. A grade of "0%" is excessive, does not change the ADHDer's future behavior (it hasn't yet, has it?), and is actually counterproductive. From a purely mathematical perspective, even getting an extra five points for extra credit on some assignments can never compensate for losing 100 points on a missed one.

Another huge benefit of these approaches is that it allows the parent to back off a little. Without the fear of a major deduction for missed work, the parent does not have to micro-manage each and every assignment—scouring everything to find that occasional missed one. That degree of parental involvement is not typically well tolerated by a teen, especially one with the low frustration threshold of ADHD. Remember that life is not all about grades. Raising a child who is grateful, moral, helpful, kind, confident, and happy is even more important. Barkley (2013, p.290) urges parents to give academics their due, but, "Do not sacrifice your parent–child relationships and emotional bonds on the altar of academic performance."

More support tips

- [ ] **Some students benefit from two sets of books.** A set of books for home, as well as a set of books to keep at school, will eliminate many stressful trips back to school to pick up textbooks.

- [ ] **Create a tangible record.** ADHD students often have an inflated sense of how well they are doing. A tangible record will allow a reality check for the child and parents.

- [ ] **Consider giving a brief pre-test** to allow for a reality test of their mastery *before* doing poorly on the test.

Use *tangible methods* to externalize problem areas.

- [ ] **Explicitly state out loud the problem and consequences** at the time of the event.

- [ ] **Use timers and planners to break down tasks into manageable, concrete chunks.** Timers give a tangible face to the nebulous concept of time, and will also help keep you from nagging. A particularly useful visual timer is available at www.timetimer. com. Personal and classroom size versions are available.

☐ *Brainstorm ideas on index cards or word processor.* Then, physically sort through and put the topics in order. Computer/tablet based graphic organizers can be found at www.inspiration.com.

☐ *Provide help for deficits at the moment it is needed*, not negative feedback when it is already too late. Unfortunately, the simple reality is that punishment does not usually teach the needed behaviors to ADHD kids. The "sink or swim" approach works poorly with ADHD. Without enabling, they will keep sinking. That helps no one.

☐ *Use the resource room or a classroom aide to give skills support* for classified children. Just teaching the skill a few dozen times to the ADHD student is not sufficient. After all, if it were sufficient, we would not still be considering these students for a skills program. The skills teacher should check organization skills daily.

» Check the assignment sheet (which will need to be checked against the web by skills teacher or parent; or, perhaps, check that a peer has initialed each assignment).

» Review books needed.

» Review due dates.

» Review plan for breaking down larger projects into steps.

» Review monthly calendar.

» The skills teacher should also check for class notes for each subject in the binder daily. Printers may be needed in skills class for those students who take notes by computer.

☐ *Keep it up.* Once a program starts to work, then the problem "no longer exists," and everyone stops doing it. People may confuse the success of the program with the lack of need for it. ("Why should I check Johnny's homework when he hasn't missed any for weeks?") Unfortunately, the same problems will tend to reoccur as soon as the support is withdrawn. By analogy, I've been successfully wearing my glasses for about four years now. My success with my glasses doesn't mean I no longer need them.

☐ *Limit non-educational "screen time"* to no more than two hours a day, according to the American Academy of Pediatrics. Currently, US children and teens spend seven hours a day using various forms of media. Besides being an incredible black hole of time, couch potato screen watching is fueling the obesity epidemic. The Academy also suggests avoid putting TV sets and internet connections in the child or teen's room (Strasburger 2011).

Further details of a school organizational system, organizing the morning and evening routines—along with teaching children how to read, take notes, and study effectively—can be found in the author's book *Organizing the Disorganized Child* (Kutscher and Moran 2009).

Feedback for physicians (if on medication)

The largest multimodal treatment trial on ADHD showed that most community-based physicians do not provide optimal medication doses (Jensen *et al.* 2001). Improved feedback from the schools would help identify areas where further improvement is still possible. Evaluations need to be done on a child's performance in different subjects at different times of the day. Teachers may submit:

☐ *a published ADHD checklist* (such as the Connor's or Vanderbilt checklist), which provides quick feedback

☐ *a written brief paragraph on the child's progress* by each teacher, which I find extremely useful.

Medication treatment for ADHD

For preschoolers, in particular, parent training and behavioral approaches are typically tried before medications, which generally do not work as well in the preschool age range.

In addition to the above, though, many children with ADHD benefit from medication. Often, medication will provide the basic neurological skills needed in order to comply with behavioral approaches. When prescribed for people who have ADHD, they stimulate the frontal parts of the brain that are not inhibiting ("filtering out") distractions as well as they should. The medications work in a similar way to caffeine. After coffee break, secretaries stop chatting and sit typing quietly, because they are now awake and alert. They don't say to each other, "You know, Jill, that coffee made me so zonked that I have no energy left to chat, so I'm just going to sit here and type quietly." No, secretaries after coffee, and people after stimulant medication, appear "calmer" because they are more alert and focused, not because they are sedated.

Unfortunately, many people do not distinguish between stimulants and sedatives. An analogy may help. Imagine that ADHD people are like bicycles without brakes. Stimulants are analogous to giving the bike new brake linings—creating a higher functioning bike. Sedatives would be like pouring tar on the gears—creating a bike that is too tired to bother anyone. Indeed, pouring tar on the gears would be horrible; but creating a properly functioning system is appropriate. Then, we can ask the ADHD person to perform correctly.

In real life, too, we know that people with ADHD are at higher risk for motor vehicle accidents and driving infractions. Stimulants have been shown to significantly reduce some of that risk. Detailed information on medications, including their benefit in driving, is given in Chapter 14.

Non-pharmacological treatments for ADHD

Unfortunately, non-pharmacological treatments for ADHD don't fare very well when subjected to blinded studies (where neither doctor nor patient knows if they are getting the actual treatment or a "placebo"). A review of the literature conducted by the European ADHD Guidelines Group showed that any positive effects on ADHD that were seen with cognitive training, neurofeedback, and food exclusions were lost when only blinded studies were included. Only omega-3/omega-6 fatty acids, and (in rare cases) elimination of food colorings in cases involving food-sensitive individuals had statistically significant—but small—effects. The analysis included 7 studies of restricted elimination diets, 8 studies of artificial food color exclusions, 11 studies of omega fatty acids, 8 neurofeedback trials, 6 studies of cognitive training and 15 behavioral interventions. The authors concluded that further evidence of efficacy of these interventions is needed before they can be recommended (Sonuga-Barke 2013). Another review concluded that although widely used, no complementary or alternative medicine met American Academy of Pediatrics criteria for evidence-based treatment, but essential fatty acids may play a small role (Bader 2012). Omega-3 fatty acids showed beneficial effect in only two out of ten studies, but combining them all into one big meta-analysis, they showed about one-third of the effectiveness of stimulant medications, and were deemed as options for families who decline traditional medications or as add-on when typical medications are not quite sufficient (Bloch and Qawasmi 2011). The verdict on neurofeedback is still up in the air, although quite costly and time intensive.

"Will it all be okay?"

Still other problems crop up as the ADHDer matures:

- being retained a grade

- less schooling

- lower salary

- higher rate of divorce

- higher frequency of driving accidents and license suspensions

- higher risk of substance abuse by 50%; we'll see in Chapter 14 on medication that stimulant medications help driving, and not only don't increase the risk of future substance abuse in ADHDers, but may even reduce it (Klein 2012).

Thus, we miss the point when we address only the triad of inattention, impulsivity, and hyperactivity. These symptoms are only the tip of the iceberg. Much greater problems have usually been plaguing the child's life, but often no one has understood that the associated symptoms described above are part and parcel of the same neurologically based condition—or are from another part of the syndrome mix. Without this recognition, caregivers have thought that their ADHD child also was "incidentally" uncooperative and apparently self-absorbed. Unless we recognize that these extended symptoms are part of the same spectrum, teachers and parents will not mention them; and doctors will never deal with them.

Given all of this, it is reasonable to ask, "Will this go away?" Fortunately, the physical hyperactivity almost always resolves by middle school. We never see a 60-year-old man jump out of a shopping cart. Without the accompanying hyperactivity, though, it's easy to misinterpret the remaining symptoms as laziness or meanness. Unfortunately, these other aspects of ADHD may persist into adulthood: although one-third of people with childhood ADHD remit by age 25, that leaves two-thirds who will continue to meet at least partial criteria, while one-sixth will continue to meet full criteria (Biederman *et al.* 2006). It's not clear, however, how much "improvement" is real versus how poorly standard criteria have applied to adults.

Personally, I would rephrase the question "Will this go away?" with "Will it all be okay?" The answer can be "yes," but we must recognize that this is often the "50-year plan" of works in progress. In other words, these children can be wonderfully successful adults, while they continue to work on these issues over their lifetime. Meanwhile, we "just" need to patiently steer them in the positive direction. If we cannot keep their self-esteem up, though, they will never productively use all of their energy when they become adults.

Finally, we must also keep in mind that some of the iceberg is fantastic and enviable. While the rest of us are obsessing about the future, or being morose about the past, people with ADHD are experiencing the present. ADHDers can be a lot of fun; dullness is never a problem. Their "why not?" attitude may free them to take chances that the rest of us may be afraid to take. Their flux of ideas may lead to creative innovations. And most importantly, their extreme passion can be a source of inspiration and accomplishment to the benefit of us all. ADHD is *part* of whom they are—a part that is responsible for many of their strengths.

It's going to be quite a ride. Let's celebrate the participants along the way!

CHAPTER 4

Specific Learning Disorders (LDs)

Robert R. Wolff, MD and Martin L. Kutscher, MD

"If I'm so smart, how come I'm in that reading group?"

Learning about learning disorders

What is "intelligence"?

What is "intelligence"? If forced to come up with a quick answer, most of us would reply, "I don't really know, but it's some kind of 'spark' that you either have or not."

However, there is no single spark that defines intelligence. Each of us has abilities in a multitude of different areas. We have separate sparks for the skills of reading (and for each of the multiple skills that go into that task), math, writing, spelling, music, art, sports, dancing, planning for the future, organization, being nice to people, saying "no" to drugs, street smarts, etc.

Even a person's "IQ" (intelligence quotient—by which most people mean the mathematically derived score on the WISC (Wechsler Intelligence Scale for Children) IQ test) actually samples 16 or so different kinds of intelligences—a set of intellectual skills needed to succeed in school. These tests are then just averaged to come up with a convenient but over-simplified single number. More details about the IQ are given at the end of this chapter.

The "spark" that is commonly considered most important in intelligence is the ability to make novel connections from previously unrelated data—a task often referred to as "creativity." We must remember, though, that this is just one of the tasks that a human being is required to do and that even this skill of making novel connections varies depending on the subject area at hand.

Defining learning disorders using simple words

All of us have some variation in our profile of these intellectual skills. For most of us, the profile would look like the rolling hills of New England. For a person with learning disorders (LDs), though, the profile would look more like the jagged Rocky Mountain landscape. Most of the skill areas are okay; but then, suddenly, a specific skill drops off of the cliff. The valleys may be identified as learning differences or, if more severe, as learning disorders. On the WISC, a difference of more than 15 points between the Performance IQ and the Verbal IQ is considered significant.

To the neurologist, a student can be considered to have areas of learning difficulty and yet have no skill below grade average. For example, if a fifth grader generally performs at a ninth grade level, and his math skills are at the sixth grade level, then his math skills will hold back his other skills—even though his weakest area is still above average.

"Learning disorder" implies an *uneven* learning profile. If the bulk of your sparks are below normal, then you are below normal intelligence (previously called "mentally retarded" and now called Intellectual Disability in DSM-5)—although such people are often euphemistically labeled as LD. In addition, a learning disorder must significantly affect the child's functioning. Dr. Betty Osman concludes that a learning disability is "a handicapping condition that interferes with the ability to store, process, or produce desired information" (Osman 1997, p.5).

No one skill defines your intellect. Being poor in the single skill of reading doesn't make you "stupid," any more than being great in the single skill of penmanship makes you a "genius."

Depending on the definition, estimates for the prevalence rate of LD in US students are about 5% (e.g., Feinstein and Phillips 2004, p.352), with estimates ranging from 1% to 10%. In general, boys are affected more commonly than girls. Learning disorders are highly inheritable. A first-degree relative of a person with a reading disorder is four to eight times more likely to have a reading disorder than a control group, and those with a mathematics disorder are five to ten times more likely to have a mathematics disorder (APA 2013, p.72).

Defining learning disorders using big words

The US federal government "legally" defines learning disabilities as follows:

> Specific learning disability means a disorder in one or more of the basic psychological processes involved in understanding or in using language, spoken or written, which may manifest itself in an imperfect ability to listen, think, speak, read, write, spell, or to do mathematical calculations. The term includes such conditions as perceptual handicaps, brain injury, minimal brain dysfunction, dyslexia, and developmental aphasia. The term does not include children who have problems that are primarily the result of visual, hearing, or motor disabilities or mental retardation, emotional disturbance, or of environmental, cultural, or economic disadvantage. (Federal law 94-142, as amended in 1977 by the Individuals with Disabilities Education Disability Act)

Defining "specific learning disorder" using DSM-5 criteria

The diagnostic term "learning disability" has now been replaced in DSM-5 by "Specific Learning Disorder." The federal government, psychologists, and school districts may have their own definitions, but the American Psychiatric Association "medically" requires specific learning disorders to meet the following summarized DSM-5 diagnostic criteria (APA 2013):

- Problem(s) with the learning and use of at least one of the academic skills below, even though interventions have been tried.

- Performance in those area(s) is substantially below expectation with resultant significant functional impairment.

- Problems began in school age, although may not become apparent until demands exceed those skills.

- Difficulties exceed those expected with any associated environmental, sensory, intellectual, or other impairment.

All learning disorders now begin with the heading "specific learning disorder," followed by specifying one of the three academic domains below, followed by specifying the problematic subskills within that domain, followed by specifying the degree of severity. The three academic domains and their subskills are:

1. with impairment in reading (can also be termed "dyslexia"):

   - word reading accuracy

   - reading rate or fluency

   - reading comprehension

2. with impairment in written expression:

   - spelling accuracy

   - grammar and punctuation accuracy

   - clarity or organization of written expression

3. with impairment in mathematics (can also be termed "dyscalculia"):

   - number sense

   - memorization of arithmetic facts

- accurate or fluent calculation

- accurate math reasoning.

So, for example, a child who has a moderate problem in math due to mathematical reasoning would have the DSM-5 diagnosis written as:

> Specific learning disorder with impairment in mathematics, with impairment in accurate math reasoning, of moderate severity.

As we shall continue to see, many of the DSM-5 formal diagnoses enable conditions to be defined much more specifically than just labeling the condition with terms such as "dyscalculia," but this comes at the expense of brevity. At the time of this writing, exactly how the new DSM-5 conventions will actually be documented and termed at meetings remains to be played out. Can you imagine parents—or nearly anybody—talking to each other with all of those helpful but wordy terms?

Developmental coordination disorder (including dysgraphia)

There is also a separate "developmental coordination disorder," in which difficulties with the skills of muscle control result in the impairment of the learning processes of writing, drawing, and sports. This disorder may be heralded by marked delays in achieving motor milestones (e.g., sitting, crawling, walking), dropping things, and "clumsiness." DSM-5 goes on with the following disclaimers: the skill deficits must be deficient for age, cause significant functional problems, begin early (although typically not formally diagnosed before age five), and not be due to something else. DSM-5 technically classifies developmental coordination disorder under the heading of "Motor Disorders," but I include it in this chapter due to it typically effecting school performance. Dysgraphia—trouble with handwriting—falls under this category. Developmental coordination disorder affects

5–6% of 5–11-year-olds, affects boys more than girls, and persists at least partially 50–70% of the time (APA 2013, pp.75–76).

When should learning disorders be identified?

Clearly, learning disorders should be identified as soon as possible. Early detection takes advantage of the brain's "plasticity," whereby the brain continues to lay down new neuronal pathways even after the child's birth. Early detection and treatment may also prevent problems with self-esteem and avoidance behaviors. Often, there are clues as early as when the child is at preschool.

Early warning signs

As we have seen, the first "red flag" should occur even before the child is born: a family history of a learning disorder, especially in a first-degree relative (parent or sibling), puts the child at significant risk. Such children should be screened carefully, including looking for the following signs, which, in general, will be evident by kindergarten or first grade. The first sign of a learning disorder may be delayed development in speech and language skills. These problematic skills may be in receptive language, processing skills, expressive language, or verbal fluency. The child may have trouble with word recall (e.g., "You know, those things that we put on our hands when it's cold out"). There may be incorrect use of prepositions (e.g., "Get that yucky food *on* my plate!"). Children with delays in language processing may understand the individual words, but they come at them so quickly that much of the message is lost. Dr. Osman (1997) likens this to the experience of traveling through a foreign country with limited skills in that language. In addition, early language problems may signify a problem with phonetics, which will later rear its head during reading decoding.

Often, learning disorders will present as avoidance or a "lack of interest" in certain tasks. For example, kids with coordination problems may veer away from writing, coloring, or drawing tasks. All of us are naturally drawn to skills that we are good at, and avoid tasks that make us feel as if we are poor performers.

Like the other disorders in this book, these problems are not the child's fault. They didn't ask for them anymore than you did. It is doubtful that any child ever woke up and consciously decided to deliberately avoid a task—just for the pleasures of never developing that skill, getting poor grades, and annoying their teachers and parents. In short, consider the possibility of LD whenever you find yourself saying, "She isn't good at it because she doesn't practice." Poor reading skills are the root cause of reading avoidance—not vice versa. That's not to say, though, that improvement doesn't require lots of practice.

Impact of learning disorders

Children with learning disorders often suffer, both in the short term and long term.

In the short term, they may not even realize that they have a specific problem. All that they know is that they are not performing well in school. Certainly by first grade, children with LD are aware that they are not performing as well as their classmates. They can identify who is in the good reading group, and who is in the poor reading group.

Even if they are assured that it is just an isolated reading problem, they can still be heard to say, "If I'm so smart, how come I can't read?" The concept of individual sparks of intelligence is hard enough for us adults to understand, much less for a first grader.

LD kids are, in essence, doing poorly at their job (learning). Imagine how you would feel if you looked around and were doing the worst job out of everybody at the office. Would you want to go to work? Imagine your frustration if you had the "Teflon syndrome," where learned material just did not stick. Teachers, themselves, may have a hard enough time handling the "Teflon syndrome" in their students. How would you handle it if you were just a little kid?

Loss of self-esteem from learning problems may lead to negative behaviors. The child may act out or become the class clown, and get sent to the principal's office. At least, there, he isn't having his nose rubbed in the fact that he cannot do the work.

Getting sent out of class is remarkably effective in the short term, even if it is a horrendous long-term strategy. Remember, though, that children are not known for their foresight.

In the long run, LD is associated with the risk for multiple problems, such as:

- poor academic achievement

- poor self-esteem, depression, anxiety, alienation, and rebellion

- other neuropsychiatric conditions of the syndrome mix covered in this book, such as a 20% risk of attention deficit hyperactivity disorder (ADHD)

- delinquency

- dropping out of school

- substance abuse—one study found 24% of students with a learning disorder had a substance abuse disorder versus 9% of non-learning disordered students (Feinstein and Phillips 2004)

- conduct disorder—85% of juvenile delinquents have received a diagnosis of learning disability (Feinstein and Phillips 2004).

Learning that life isn't always fair is a tough lesson.

Try some of the simulations of learning disorders at our website www.pediatricneurology.com/adhd2.htm. The frustration that you experience from these simulations may increase your empathy for the child with LD.

Supporting the child with learning disorders and differences

General approaches

Academic skills are important, but they are only potential vehicles to a greater goal: a life filled with enough self-worth and happiness that you can help someone else reach those same goals of self-worth and happiness. Our goal as a child's caregiver is to maximize his potential as he moves along this path. Reading well is important; being happy and helpful is more important.

There are two basic types of strategies to help children move along this path.

1. Strategies that "hammer away" at the area of deficit.

2. Strategies that effectively circumvent or accommodate it.

In dyslexia, for example, Orton-Gillingham (a structured, multi-sensory approach, stressing phonics grounded on language-based learning processes) is the hammer-away approach, whereas using books on tape is the circumvent approach. Both types of interventions have their essential and legitimate uses.

As Dr. Osman points out, sometimes it might be better to consider learning disorders as "learning differences." Reframing the "problem" as a "difference" causes us to seek alternate strengths that are different but work to help circumvent/overcome the weaknesses (Osman 1997, p.8). For example, if a child has an auditory processing problem, it is helpful to ask ourselves, "What *different* learning strategies *would* work?" In this case, we might remind ourselves that extensive use of the blackboard would help the child understand the material.

Homework suggestions for children with LD

In her book *Learning Disabilities and ADHD*, Dr. Betty Osman (1997) offers the following homework rules to be shared by teachers and parents.

1. Showing/helping a child with the homework is better than letting him agonize through it by himself. The child may really not have understood or paid attention to the class instruction. Agony that bears no fruit just leads to further avoidance.

2. For children with learning disabilities, it will typically take several explanations and reviews of the material to master it.

3. Break assignments into smaller pieces. For example, when reading a chapter, start by looking at the questions at the end, and find the answer to each question before reading the entire chapter. Many students still need to be taught how to study!

4. It is okay for the parent to be the secretary until the child becomes competent enough to readily handle the whole process by himself. (See the following section on use of word processors.)

5. Similarly, the parent may help a child by copying math problems if that proves to be the difficulty.

6. Make sure the student understands the directions *before* she does the work.

7. Start the first few problems together.

8. Pre-teach the material for the next day. Be aware, though, that many children are not interested in learning anything that is not required to enter class the next day. Dads, in particular, seem to need to keep this in mind.

9. Don't worry about the child becoming dependent on the parent as a crutch. Most children will give it up as soon as they can. (More typically, parents have trouble getting the kid to accept the help in the first place.)

10. If a child accepts a parent's help, then fine. Otherwise, get outside help.

Be sure to keep the teachers in the loop of how you are helping—otherwise they'll think the child is fine and won't be aware of the need for their further support during school.

Word processors

For many students with learning disorders, ready access to a word processor is essential. The goal is to get the typist up and running quickly. Many students can start effective keyboarding by third grade, and research studies have started as early as first grade. There are many enticing computer games to learn typing at home. If possible, the child would ideally learn to use all ten fingers, but we'll settle for whatever works. It is okay if they look at their hands while typing. After all, there is no handwritten rough draft that they need to keep their eyes on. Once students have learned basic comfort on the keyboard, then homework and the internet will provide the needed practice.

The advantages of using a word processor are numerous.

- It helps with dysgraphia, freeing the child's mind to focus on ideas rather than letter formations.

- Spell check and grammar check are lifesavers. Don't worry—the child still has to decide which correct spelling to use. Let's just hope we can get them to look at those squiggly red and green lines.

- Learning to use a word processor is a life skill. There will be very little serious written work in a child's future that does not include one. All they really need to do by hand in the future is sign their name. When's the last time you wrote out anything important by hand? What do college professors expect?

- The ability to easily make corrections will encourage the child to accept editing suggestions from the parent/ teacher, since that does not mean copying the whole thing over.

- Quick future editing may make it easier for children with writer's block. They just need to start typing something. They can come back later for corrections.

- For pre-typists, parental use of a word processor lets the child focus on the more important aspects of the assignment. If a child has a writing problem, then consider having the child write what he can in the amount of time that the assignment is expected to take, and then let him dictate the rest to the parent. It is better to learn how to tell a creative story than it is to suffer through dysgraphia.

A few caveats on the use of computers:

- Elementary school teachers may be uncomfortable with the use of a word processor in class. The bell rings, the child runs out, and now the teacher is left feeling responsible for this expensive machine sitting in the middle of the classroom. In this setting, a good compromise is to allow the child to practice handwriting in class and typing at home.

- The school may consider a simple word-processing machine or netbook to be appropriate, rather than a full-fledged notebook computer.

- Students may feel stigmatized by the use of a word processor. This often resolves by secondary school. We can only push the child so far.

- The child's homework station should be equipped with its own computer and printer. It is not reasonable to expect a child with homework/ADHD problems to go back and forth between multiple work areas.

- No games or unmonitored/uncontrolled internet connection should be on the child's laptop. They are much too distracting. Be aware that games seem to have their own mysterious habit of apparently loading themselves onto a child's computer.

Specific learning disorders

Reading disorder ("dyslexia")

"Dyslexia" simply denotes abnormal reading. Of all learning disorders, reading dysfunction has the most significant educational impact. Practically all subjects in school require reading proficiency, including math word problems, and science. Although many people may focus on dyslexia as letter reversals, that is not typically the case. *Reading disorders reflect a problem with phonics.* About 10% of children have some degree of dyslexia (Feinstein and Phillips 2004).

Steps involved in reading

DSM-5 breaks down dyslexia into impairment of any/all of three skills:

1. word reading accuracy

2. reading rate or fluency

3. reading comprehension.

We'll combine the first two under "decoding" and add another skill of "retention."

Thus, in order to understand dyslexia, we need to consider three major steps in reading, which include:

1. decoding

2. comprehension

3. retention.

Decoding is the first step. Research clearly shows that phonological dysfunction is the root problem for most people who have trouble deciphering the written word. Dyslexic children start by having trouble breaking down ("deconstructing") words into their basic *phonemes*. Phonemes are the smallest elements of sound that make up words. For example, the word "this" has three phonemes blended together: th—i—s. We are wired to understand the sounds of phonemes. Note that the brain's comprehension center is not neurologically programmed to understand squiggly black lines and curves (written letters). An understanding of the system of sounds of speech is a prerequisite to recognizing the sounds that a written letter codes for. In other words, first a child needs to learn phonemic awareness (being aware of and manipulating the sounds of language) and then learn the system of phonics (how letter symbols code for those sounds of speech) in school (Shaywitz 2003, p.262). This is why reading is an academic skill that needs to be formally taught in school, while speech develops naturally.

Delays in speech, insensitivity to rhyme, and trouble with articulation (particularly after five to six years of age) may be early warning signs of phonetic difficulties and impending dyslexia. Later, trouble attaching names to letters in kindergarten (e.g., "That's the letter *K*") and trouble attaching sounds to letters (e.g., "*K* is for *kite*") by late kindergarten/early first grade, are huge red flags of underlying problems. Early phonologic problems are a sign of reading difficulties, and should trigger an automatic referral for assessment. However, despite the difficulty that dyslexic children have in labeling letters, "there is no evidence that they actually *see* letters and words backwards" (Shaywitz 2003, p.100). Visual tracking is *not* felt to be a typical problem in dyslexia. Most objective authorities agree that visual exercises are of no help in dyslexia and may take time away from other more effective strategies.

You should pay attention to reading automaticity and fluency. By the middle of first grade, reading should be no more "work" than speaking. Some children can read but it is too "effortful" to maintain. Since their decoding skills are frail and inconsistent, they come across each word as if seeing it for the first time. Research shows that a child must *consistently and accurately* experience a word at least four times in order for it to become neurologically automatic and thus a fluent part of the child's reading. This repetition should be done with familiar texts and out loud so that an adult can provide corrective (yet supportive) feedback. Otherwise, it's like forever seeing the word for the first time—sounding it out and attaching meaning to it yet again. Remember, having a dysfluent child merely read silently to herself doesn't do the trick.

Unfortunately, it has been my experience that many reading achievement tests fail to detect effortfulness. I feel like telling the Committee of Special Education at the school, "Just listen to her read for one minute a passage she hasn't seen before, and then tell me if her reading isn't difficult for her!" As Sally Shaywitz—a leading Yale neuroscientist and researcher on dyslexia—says, "A child who reads accurately but not fluently is dyslexic" (2003, p.133).

Reading comprehension problems may be due to early decoding problems, as so much effort is spent on breaking the phonics code that little brainpower is left to understand what was just read. However, reading comprehension problems can also occur without reading decoding difficulties. The child might whiz through the passage, but have no clue as to its literal or deeper/inferential meaning. They might gloss over important details, may be unable to distinguish important from unimportant facts, may not be able to see the connections between facts, or simply not understand words or sentences.

Retention problems may also exist. By third grade, "reading to learn" (versus "learning to read," which is the focus of early elementary years) is an essential part of amassing information. Early signs of reading retention problems include trouble recalling or summarizing what was just read, or connecting it to previous knowledge or personal experiences.

Importance of early detection and aggressive treatment

A series of review articles (Torgesen 2004; Wattenberg 2004) in the Fall 2004 issue of *American Educator* (the quarterly journal of the American Federation of Teachers) makes the following essential points:

- The "late bloomer" theory of reading lag is officially dead; 88% of poor readers at the end of first grade will still be poor readers at the end of fourth grade—unless there is early, aggressive intervention.

- Left to their own devices, poor readers will fall further behind. Dyslexia is not a temporary lag. Untreated, it is a chronic condition.

- Reading problems are typically due to deficits in phonics skills.

- Poor, inconsistent decoding skills hinder development of essential sight-word recognition. Good readers develop a much larger library of sight-words than do poor readers.

- Poor decoding skills means poor vocabulary development.

- Poor decoding skills lead to poor comprehension skills.

- All of the above lead to lack of practice in reading— by just the children who actually need extra practice. This lack of practice prevents the repeated exposure to words that is needed for automaticity to develop.

- Recognize the red flags of reading problems. According to Schatschneider and Torgesen (2004), the following problems should lead to further evaluation, monitoring, and likely treatment:

  - Failure to know the names of letters by early kindergarten.

  - Failure to know the sounds of letters by late kindergarten.

  - Trouble with decoding and reading fluency by the second part of first grade.

- Early detection is essential. Students from kindergarten to third grade should be repeatedly screened formally and informally.

- Although many children are not identified as being dyslexic until third grade or later, that is too late: *wiring of the brain for reading winds down after third grade.* Progress after that is much slower. (This is analogous to learning a foreign language, which involves effortlessly laying down new brain wiring by a young child, but is much more labored and slow in an adult.) Additionally, later diagnosis leaves a bigger gap of unread words for the child to make up, and may also lead to loss of self-esteem and interest in school (Shaywitz 2003, p.30).

- Aggressive and early treatment is successful for most children. Depending on the particular study of early, intensive intervention, 56–92% of poor readers have been brought into the average range. This hopefully includes starting by kindergarten and first grade.

- Early intervention is much more successful than later treatment.

- Children identified as at-risk for reading problems need reading instruction that is:

  ○ *more explicit* than for other students (no decoding skill can be taken for granted. The connection between a letter and its sound should be taught in a comprehensive fashion. Words and their associated meanings need to be explicitly taught)

  ○ *more intensive* than for other students (typically, this would mean time in small groups—which allows for individualization and the required feedback needed by the student)

  ○ *more supportive* than for other students (the appropriate scaffolding of basic skills needs to be steady before taking on the next step. Positive reinforcement is essential)

  ○ *integrated with the curriculum* being taught in the regular classroom.

According to Sally Shaywitz (2003, p.28), reading programs should not just be aimed at those students who meet some arbitrary cut-off. Rather, since research shows that dyslexia is a continuum, not a discrete entity, borderline readers should receive support as well. In fact, since their problem is less severe, they are most likely to benefit from explicit phonics support.

The above general guidelines may need to be adjusted to the individual child and school district. It is important to note that each state and district in the US has its own teaching style mandates.

Treatment approaches for the regular classroom teacher

The regular classroom teacher can use the following suggestions to supplement the additional individualized interventions:

☐ *Phonics will be essential for the poor decoder.* Although 70–80% of US school children can learn phonics relatively easily, that leaves 20–30% who need greater phonics support. We cannot assume that everyone can teach themselves the rules of phonics.

☐ *The entire class would benefit from a systematic, scientifically validated, phonics based approach to reading.* Suggestions for such programs can be found in Shaywitz (2003).

☐ *Sight-word recognition should be taught* for words that do not follow the phonic rules, and for speed.

The following list of suggestions for helping students with reading problems is largely inspired by Dr. Kenneth Shore's excellent book *Special Kids Problem Solver* (2002).

☐ *If a child does not read very often, check if there is a problem.* Ask the child to read out loud for you in private. Can he read phonetically, blend sounds, and comprehend what he read? When in doubt, have the child checked by the school's reading specialist. Formal and informal screenings are ideally repeated through the early school years.

☐ *Teach phonics,* starting at the beginning if needed. You may need to start over with letter formation, letter sounds, and blending sounds. Use materials that allow these skills to be practiced in the context of *meaningful* material. This will often require a small group setting.

☐ *Provide individualized sessions* for special needs students to go over the material.

☐ *Reading, reading, everywhere.* Point out that words are everywhere: T-shirts, greetings cards, signs, posters, magazines, and books. Have books of all levels and many areas of interest easily accessible in the room. Try to have material of interest to the child.

☐ *Give reading material at a level that encourages a sense of mastery.* In order for a text to be enjoyable, the child should be able to read at least 90% of the words with relative ease and accuracy. Give material based on the child's ability, not his chronological age. Re-reading material adds to the sense of success and builds the automaticity required for fluency. *Do not frustrate the child!*

☐ *Use multisensory approaches.* Have the student say the letter while drawing it with his finger in the air, in the sand, in his mind, or in finger-paint. The goal is to see, hear, and touch the letters.

☐ *Encourage the child to visualize* the scene that the words describe.

☐ *Teach to sight read commonly used words.* This will speed up reading. The first 100 words of Fry's Instant Word List make up 50% of a student's reading. These words can be placed on a "word wall," and five words a week can be practiced. Download the list from www.makereadingfirst.com/word_list.pdf.

☐ *Lessen the stress of reading out loud.* Allow the student to practice the passage in advance, do not correct minor mistakes in the mainstream class, and make sure no one ever criticizes. If necessary, allow the student to skip this task.

☐ *Utilize books on tape* to familiarize the child with the material he will read.

☐ *Keep reading to the child.* Let him know that there is great stuff waiting in all of those books.

☐ *Teach and model comprehension strategies,* such as how to:

  » pre-read the text quickly; this allows the student to know where the text is going, and gives a framework upon which to hang the new information

  » ask questions and/or make predictions about what will happen next

  » convert textbook topic headings into questions. For example, change the topic heading "The Causes of World War II" into the question, "What were the causes of WWII?" Now, you are reading that section with a purpose

  » ask yourself questions about what you just read, and answer them(!)

  » monitor your own comprehension, to determine when you need to slow down or re-read a passage

  » summarize what you just read

  » read out loud, if needed, to help comprehension (although that certainly slows reading).

☐ *Provide reading aid in advance,* for example:

  » go over difficult words in the passage

  » give a summary, or even an outline

  » construct a visual map of the information to show how it all connects.

☐ *DEAR* (Drop Everything And Read) time. Give the class 20 minutes per day of high-priority, uninterrupted silent reading time. Make it a daily highlight and treat.

☐ *Encourage parents to read to their young child every day.* Make it a special time.

☐ *Work with the school reading specialist or psychologist.*

☐ *Keep it fun!*

Celebrate the unique strengths that often accompany dyslexia

Shaywitz (2003, p.53) urges us to continue to celebrate the children's strengths, which is a recurrent theme in taking care of special kids. In dyslexia, these strengths often include complex reasoning and sophisticated thinking skills—as well as the ability to think out of the box—since they may need to practice higher order thinking skills in order to get around their phonetic block. People with:

> dyslexia appear to be disproportionately represented in the upper echelons of creativity and in the people who, whether in business, finance, medicine, writing, law, or science, have broken through a boundary and have made a real difference to society. I believe that this is because a dyslexic cannot simply memorize or do things by rote, she must get far underneath the concept and understand it at a fundamental level. (Shaywitz 2003, p.57)

Unfortunately, this circuitous route to understanding takes more time than it does for a fluent reader, leading to the need for accommodations.

Accommodations for dyslexia

Most of the above support can be carried out by an understanding teacher without the student being formally classified by the school. The following additional accommodations may be under a school's "504" or "IEP." (Readers can find information about terms such as "504," "IDEA," and "IEP" at www.ldonline.org and www.wrightslaw.com.) These *accommodations* become even more important as the student enters middle school and above (whereas *prevention and remediation/differentiated instruction services* predominate in the early school years). They provide the bridge for the child to access and demonstrate her higher level thinking skills.

☐ ***Extra time on exams is essential*** for dyslexic children. Children with dyslexia can understand; it just takes more time.

☐ ***Exams should be held in quiet locations,*** as the student's reading skills are tenuous and require intense concentration.

☐ ***Avoid multiple-choice questions.*** These are notoriously difficult for dyslexic children, as they are require intense reading, yet do not give enough context for the child to understand what she is reading. Use oral or essay exams instead.

☐ ***Shorten the length of assignments.*** The children (and their parents) have lives to live!

☐ ***Equip children with notes*** from the teacher, a peer, or a scribe.

☐ ***Use a laptop for spelling/grammar.*** Minimize or eliminate penalties for misspelling.

☐ ***Use other technology and computer programs,*** such as books on tape, scanners that read books, magazines, etc. out loud while the student follows along. There are word processors that offer the student definitions of homonyms (such as *meat* and *meet*) so that he can choose/learn the one with the right meaning (see Shaywitz 2003). The Live Scribe pen (www.livescribe.com) records the teacher while the student takes notes on special paper with microscopic dots on it. To hear playback of what the teacher actually said at that point in the notes, the student merely touches the pen to that spot on the notepad and the recording queues to that moment.

Treatment with specialized instruction

If the above interventions do not lead to clear improvements (six months should be enough time to tell), then the child needs to be formally classified, and receive differentiated instruction. A successful program should be:

- scientifically validated

- explicitly phonics based (children are not left on their own to hopefully figure it out)

- hierarchically structured and systematic (builds upon itself)

- intensive (daily) and relentless

- for a small group (maximum of four students to each special education teacher to allow for individualization and frequent feedback/correction)

- multisensory (such as having the child tap out the syllables.)

- taught by teachers who are trained in the program.

Elements to be taught should include:

- phonemic awareness (recognizing and manipulating the sounds of speech)

- phonics (how letters represent those sounds)

- decoding/spelling/comprehension

- sight words

- practice, practice, practice

- fluency work

- connecting with enriched language experiences (telling stories, etc.).

(Shaywitz 2003, p.262)

Orton-Gillingham and Wilson's reading programs seem to be the most popular in my experience, although other programs provide more comprehensive support in writing, vocabulary, and comprehension skills.

Parents must remain the child's advocate, ensuring that their child is receiving and benefiting from an appropriate program, which also brings out the child's strengths and connects with the school's regular academic program.

For more advice on all aspects of dyslexia—including its underpinnings, early identification, early and later treatment at home and at school, accommodations, school placement, and further resources—the author strongly recommends Sally Shaywitz's superb book, *Overcoming Dyslexia: A New and Complete Science-Based Program for Reading Problems at any Level* (2003).

Mathematics disorder (dyscalculia)

Early signs of a mathematics disorder include difficulty with sorting items by shape or size, or matching numbers with quantities. Typical children learn their early math calculations with visual reinforcement, such as counting fingers, but become less reliant on these as they practice. Children with a math disorder, though, may experience the "Teflon effect" as they try to master simple addition and subtraction—no less with multiplication, division, or algebra. Despite repetition, it is harder for them to make math facts automatic. Mathematics disorders are divided in DSM-5 into impairment(s) of:

- number sense
- memorization of arithmetic facts
- accurate or fluent calculation
- accurate math reasoning.

Dyscalculia occurs in 5–6% of school-age children (Shalev 2004). Some, but not all, studies show predominance amongst girls.

Treatment approaches

The following recommendations are largely based on Dr. Kate Garnett's article *Math Learning Disabilities* (1998).

TROUBLE WITH BASIC NUMBER FACTS

☐ *Give intensive practice,* with materials that gain the student's attention. Use games that motivate children to actually pay attention to their practice.

☐ *Distribute practice in multiple, short sessions* (about 15 minutes each).

☐ *Master small groups of calculations at a time.* Then mix the different groups.

☐ *Teach special sets of problems,* such as 5+5, 6+6, 7+7 or 5+6, 6+7, 7+8...

☐ *Use accommodative strategies.*

　　» Use a calculator.

　　» Use personal math fact summary charts (pocket sized). Block off answers as they are mastered.

☐ *Keep a child who has good math concepts in a stimulating math tract,* while simultaneously acknowledging and treating specific problem areas.

TROUBLE UNDERSTANDING MATHEMATICAL SYMBOLS

☐ *Use concrete manipulatives* along with the graphical symbols. Learning the meaning of symbols such as "–" can be difficult even for a child who naturally understands the concept of subtraction.

TROUBLE WITH THE VERBAL PARTS INVOLVED IN MATH

☐ *Break instructions into small chunks.*

☐ *Give instructions slowly.*

☐ *Have students explain the math process* to themselves or to others. Having the student teach the process helps to clarify and integrate the material.

☐ *Have students self-verbalize* what the problem is asking them to do.

☐ *For word problems, teach that "is" means "=."* For example, "John's age plus Jill's age *is* 24" means "John's age plus Jill's age = 24." Also, "of" means "x" (times). For example, "½ *of* 10 is 5" means "½ x 10 = 5."

TROUBLE WITH THE VISUAL-SPATIAL PARTS OF MATH—
COMPENSATE BY USING WORDS OR MANIPULATIVES

☐ *Use words to describe what most of us "see."* For example, most of us see something with three sides and instantly visually recognize it as a triangle. Students with visual-spatial problems may need to be told (or say to themselves): "I have counted three sides. That makes this a triangle."

☐ *Teach the child to talk himself through each step of a problem.*

☐ *Use verbal constructs* (words!) rather than diagrams.

☐ *Supplement instruction with concrete manipulatives.*

TROUBLE WITH THE GRAPHOMOTOR PARTS OF MATH

☐ *Use graph paper* to line up problems.

☐ *Encourage students to show their work in a vertical fashion,* with each step shown below the previous step.

☐ *Use lots and lots of space on handouts/homework.* Don't cram it all into tiny spaces on one page. This is no time to save trees.

Written expression disorder and dysgraphia

Writing disorders are subclassified in DSM-5 as impairment(s) of:

- spelling accuracy
- grammar and punctuation accuracy
- clarity or organization of written expression.

We include dysgraphia (handwriting problems due to a developmental coordination disorder) here, since it so frequently occurs with written expression disorder. Handwriting itself requires an orchestration of a remarkably complex sequence of movements. Writing disorders occur in some 2–8% of children, predominantly in boys (Feinstein and Phillips 2004). Usually, it occurs in combination with other disabilities, such as a reading disorder or developmental coordination disorder. Writing is even more difficult than reading. In reading, the ideas and organization are all laid out for you in advance; in writing, all you get is a blank piece of paper.

Treatment approaches

- ☐ *Liberal use of a laptop.* See the previous material on use of computers.

- ☐ *Give extra points for neatness,* but minimize deductions for messiness (i.e., keep it positive).

- ☐ *Provide the student with alternate ways of getting notes:* a copy of a peer's notes, a copy of the teacher's notes, or a scribe.

- ☐ *Consider referral to occupational therapy* for handwriting problems.

- ☐ *Teach how to organize thoughts*—utilizing graphic organizers, sorting index cards, outlining, etc. See my book, *Organizing the Disorganized Child: Simple Strategies to Succeed in School* (Kutscher and Moran 2009) for additional methods of helping writing, reading, and studying.

- ☐ *Give exams orally, or allow use of a scribe.* Remember: is the goal of this particular test to check, for example, a student's knowledge of photosynthesis, or is the goal to test writing skills? (Yes, in most students, we want to teach and test both subject knowledge and writing skills, but this is not the typical student.)

Intellectual disability (intellectual developmental disorder)—formerly called mental retardation (MR)

In contrast to children with learning disorders (who have highly variable skills), the DSM-5 diagnosis of "Intellectual Disability" (formerly called mental retardation or "MR") is the term applied when most of a person's individual sparks are well below average. There may still be variations, but overall, most intellectual skills are poor. There may sometimes be additional muscle control problems, but they are not considered part of intellectual disability, per se. Three out of every 100 people has the condition; and in most of these individuals, the degree of retardation is mild (Szymanski and Kaplan 2004). Children with autistic spectrum disorder have a higher incidence of intellectual disability, but are particularly likely to have extreme variations in their different cognitive skills.

What is "IQ"?

More formally, intellectual disability is partly quantified by IQ, which stands for intelligence quotient. If, for example, a ten-year-old child functions intellectually at the six-year-old level, then his $IQ = 6/10 = 60\% = "60."$

There are a number of IQ tests, of which we most commonly mean the Wechsler Intelligence Scale (WISC). The WISC-IV examination consists of 16 subtests, which are grouped together to derive four scores—Verbal, Perceptual, Memory, and Processing Speed. The WISC-IV has norms for children of different groups, such as ADHD, Asperger's, etc.

A "normal" IQ is considered to be in the range of 90–110, with an IQ of 100 being perfectly *average* for age. The standard deviation is 15 points. The "intellectual disability" range IQ is defined as more than two standard deviations below the norm (i.e., IQ <70 +/– 5). The first clue of a mildly low IQ is typically poor academic performance in the early primary grades. Assessment and identification are critical to determine special needs. Such children may benefit greatly from specifically directed vocational programs in secondary school.

DSM-5 criteria for intellectual disability

Here are greatly simplified medical DSM-5 criteria for intellectual disability. The child must meet all three conditions.

1. Deficits in intellectual functioning. For example, solving problems, thinking abstractly, judgment, or learning. This tends to correlate with an IQ of approximately 70 or below.

2. Trouble with adaptive functioning in at least one of these three areas of life:

   a. concepts: academic and practical knowledge

   b. social: skills of friendship and social judgment

   c. practical: personal care, job responsibilities, money management, transportation.

3. Onset before age 18.

DSM-5 uses clinical judgment to add "severity levels" of mild, moderate, severe, and profound to the diagnosis.

Although now outdated terms, the DSM-IV criteria, which used the full-scale IQ to define the following subcategories, are presented for informational and historical purposes.

- *Mild MR*—IQ range of 50–55 to approximately 70. Represents the vast majority of people with MR. Such children typically reach a sixth grade level by their late teens.

- *Moderate MR*—IQ range of 35–40 to 50–55.

- *Severe MR*—IQ range of 20–25 to 35–40.

- *Profound MR*—IQ below 20–25. These more severely affected children are more likely to have a diagnosable neurological problem. There is an increased risk of seizures, motor impairments, communication deficits; as well as psychiatric disorders including anxiety, mood disturbances, and psychosis.

The education process for children with intellectual disability

Children with intellectual disability usually appear normal initially, and have normal acquisition of gross motor and fine motor milestones (unless accompanied by another disorder), but usually show some delay in comprehending verbal concepts or immaturity of behavior. The condition is often not first appreciated until approximately four to six years of age, when they appear to be slow in processing information, and seem less capable than their peers in coping with academic challenges. Psycho-educational testing should be done for any child where such a suspicion exists in order to determine the appropriate education placement.

The education of children with intellectual disability requires a high degree of individual commitment, patience, willingness to provide emotional support, and constant repetition. Fortunately, the last several decades have witnessed a quiet but positive revolution in the care of such individuals. In contrast to the massive "warehouses" that existed for the mentally disabled not that many years ago, such children are cared for at home. Services such as speech therapy, occupational therapy, cognitive therapy, and physical therapy are now largely under the auspices of preschool, and school programs.

Inclusion programs, in which children are placed in a mainstream classroom regardless of their disability, present a particular challenge to teachers and students alike. The benefit of this controversial but widely practiced educational experiment has yet to be conclusively determined.

The educational process for children with intellectual disability requires an emphasis on training for pragmatic life skills. Unfortunately, children with such disabilities rarely acquire the ability to achieve independent citizenship. Being able to manage a bank account, read a tax form, or arrange for a mortgage may be simply beyond their capacities. They will require ongoing support services throughout life, some to a much greater degree than others.

CHAPTER 5

Autism Spectrum Disorder (ASD)

An Overview

Great, you figured out or discovered something. Congratulations! Now, you may want to share that idea with another human mind. If so, your brain translates the idea into a sequence of words. The words are translated into vibrations that depart from your mouth, sail long distances through the air, and land on my eardrum. These vibrations are turned back into words, and then into meaningful sentences and ideas. My brain also picks up other non-verbal language, such as your facial expression and tone of voice. Meanwhile, I figure out any "hidden agenda" or "subtext" when you said those words. All of these elements mix together to come up with an accurate understanding of what your "self" meant to communicate to my "self."

With this much involved, it's amazing that humans can interact fully at all. It is not really amazing that some people have trouble with some aspect of the process. Given all of the ways that communication can go awry, this is a complex topic. Note that in this chapter "communication" is used in the broadest possible sense, including spoken speech, non-verbal clues, and the ability to use imagination and symbolic representations, as well as the urge and the ability to socialize. After all, what's the purpose of communicating if it isn't to interact with others, i.e., to socialize, and, conversely, how do we socialize without communicating?

First, we'll start with a discussion of the underlying skills involved in communication, and then move on to the actual autism spectrum disorders (ASDs), exploring both the previous and newer classifications. As we pull together a lot of essential information, we'll try to demystify technical terms. Hold on to your hats!

Skills involved in communication

Communication involves two broad areas: *literal verbal skills*, and *non-verbal skills*. People with an ASD have problems that include (at a minimum) the non-verbal areas—including difficulty with their desire and/or ability to use language in a back-and-forth, social context. (They also have a restricted and/or repetitive range of interests or activities.) Let's examine these categories of communication skills in more detail.

Literal verbal/spoken communication skills

Semantic language refers to the ability to use and understand words, phrases, and sentences; including abstract concepts and idioms. These skills involved in the literal use of verbal language may or may not be affected in ASDs. The skills needed for semantic language include the following:

- *Receptive verbal language*—the ability to *understand* spoken/written words and ideas. One type of receptive language disorder involves central auditory processing (CAP), which is used to get meaning from sounds and words. Such auditory processing skills include the ability to distinguish between similar sounds, and to pick out the main voice from the background. CAP is covered in Chapter 13.

- *Expressive verbal language*—the ability to *express* our ideas with spoken/written words, including the ability to articulate each word clearly. A problem with communicating with gestures (such as signing) would also fall under the category of an expressive language disorder.

Currently DSM-5, as I understand it, gives the same name of "language disorder" to either or both receptive and expressive language problems (although I certainly intend to continue to document the different types).

Non-verbal/non-spoken communication/ socialization skills

By definition, people with ASD have problems in the non-verbal/ non-spoken areas of communication. (Note that restricted range of interests and/or repetitive behaviors interfere with socialization and are the other major part of ASD.)

Let's explain non-verbal communication by way of analogy. Imagine that a typical three-year-old, English-speaking child is parachuted into Russia. Some Russian women—who don't speak any English—find him. Even though they would not understand any words from each other, they would be able to have a great deal of communication/socialization. The child could let the women know that he was scared and hungry. The women could let him know that he was welcome, and that they'd take care of him. All of this would happen without words. It is just like if you go to a restaurant in a foreign country—everyone would know that you were enjoying the experience, even without your saying it. Similarly, a typical child who is told by a peer, "Nice job!" after striking out with the bases loaded in the ninth inning of the baseball game still can figure out that he is being insulted despite the literal meaning of the words. Such is the power of non-verbal communication.

The communicative/socialization skills that are still available to the child parachuted into a foreign country—including the desire to communicate and form a bond—are the areas that are weak in a child with an ASD. As I see it, these skills break down into two basic categories: the *urge* to socialize, and the *ability* to socialize. In summary, these skills include:

- the *urge* to initiate shared social interaction and two-way communication: theory of mind

- the *ability* to carry out that urge to socialize:
  - pragmatic language
  - knowledge of unwritten rules
  - knowing what is and isn't important
  - symbolic play skills
  - the ability to achieve "joint attention"
  - non-verbal (non-spoken) transmission of language.

Let's look at the urge and the ability to socialize in some more detail.

The urge to initiate shared social interaction and two-way communication: theory of mind

The urge to socialize/relate/empathize requires a working "theory of mind." Theory of mind refers to the relatively unique ability of humans to understand: that I have a mind; that you have a mind; and most importantly, that our minds may or may not know or be feeling the same things. Without a theory of mind, there is little point in communicating. There is limited ability to truly recognize that there is another human being in the room. It is difficult to feel the need to communicate with anyone else. After all, with whom would you be communicating? Eye contact will be poor. It may seem as if there is a pane of glass between the child and others. There may be a paucity of spontaneous speech, except when the child has a need that can only be met with the help of others.

With limited ability to "get inside your mind," it will be difficult for the child to demonstrate empathy for what you are feeling. After all, empathy is virtually defined as "putting yourself in someone else's shoes." A child with theory of mind problems may assume that since he is happy, then you must be happy; or the child may not understand that someone else is deceptive when he is always bluntly honest.

Thus, the ability to recognize that other people have a mind, the ability to relate to that mind, and the ability to empathize with that mind are all parts of the same skill. Theory of mind problems may underlie many of the difficulties seen in the autism spectrum disorders.

The ability to carry out the urge for shared social interaction

Closely related to this *urge/interest* in social communication (that arises from a working theory of mind) is the *ability* to communicate socially. The skills discussed below are required to actually achieve the meaningful interaction. Certainly, if you don't have these required skills, your interest in social interaction may appear blunted. Some children with intact social urge are painfully aware of their inability to effectively carry out that desire.

Pragmatic language

Pragmatic language is the practical ability to use language in a social setting, such as knowing what it is appropriate to say, and where and when to say it; and the give-and-take nature of conversation. Effective pragmatics requires a working theory of mind: the ability to figure out what the other person does or does not already know—or might or might not be interested in hearing about. Some examples of pragmatic language/theory of mind problems are given below.

- A new student moves into the school district and enters the classroom for the first time. The teacher asks him where he comes from. The autism spectrum child responds, "From the hallway."

- As a child with a mild ASD walks into the office, the doctor notices that her pink shirt matches the color of her jacket. He jokes, "If you change into a green shirt, does the color of the jacket change, too?" The child responds, "My wardrobe includes a turquoise shirt, not a green one." This child's spoken language is precise, but she misses that the whole purpose of this conversation was just a little fun chitchat to initiate an interaction.

Knowledge of unwritten rules

There is an incredible array of essential social norms that most typical children do not need to be explicitly taught. Did your mother have to tell you to look at people when you talk to them? Did your mother have to teach you how close to stand to someone? Did your father have to teach you how to read facial expressions?

Liane Holliday Willey describes her own frustrating experience with Asperger's as follows:

> I never got the hang of it. For example, I can never tell how much time should pass before I buy for someone I just met a "thinking of you gift." Do I really have to talk on the phone to anyone if I think the conversation is boring or a waste of my time? If there is a lapse in the conversation, am I supposed to hang up or tell a joke or just sit there? What if I like the person well enough, but I decide I cannot stand one of their behaviors or habits? The questions are endless, and the concerns are mountain high. This is why human relationships usually take me beyond my limits. They wear me out. (Willey 1999, p.55)

Unwritten rules are innate or self-taught to a typical child. They usually do not require much explicit teaching. So, as a quick rule of thumb, whenever you find yourself teaching a rule to your child while saying, "I shouldn't have to tell you that..." consider that you might be dealing with an ASD symptom.

Knowing what is and isn't important

The skills to know what is—and what isn't—important include:

- the ability to see the big picture rather than fixate on details

- the ability to maintain a full range of interests

- the ability to narrate a story with an appropriate amount of detail.

Symbolic play skills

Give a child a yellow box on wheels, with thin long black stripes on it. The ability to understand that this object actually represents a school bus is a type of communication. Speech pathologist Elaine Schneider points out that, if a child cannot even recognize that a physical toy bus stands for a real bus, how will he be able to recognize later that the graphic letters "B—U—S" represents a bus, too? Both involve the use of symbols rather than the actual object to communicate (Schneider, verbal communication 2005).

By 18 months, most toddlers start to use objects as symbols for something else. For example, a cup is for drinking, but it also makes quite a handy telephone. By three years of age, most children are quite good at "let's pretend" activities, such as "You be the cowboy!" The toy school bus is not fascinating because the cold metal box can move, but because little toy figures chat while getting on it as they go to school. Stuffed animals are not just warm rags of cloth to drag around, but appear to be living creatures that have feelings and needs such as to be fed, dressed, and loved.

So, by 18–36 months of age, typical children make continuous progress in the skill of appreciating the representational meaning of a toy, rather than focusing on its straightforward physical attributes. Spectrum children tend to have more mechanical play, such as lining, sorting, dumping, or watching things spin. Failure to develop representational/symbolic/pretend play is a strong marker of the autism spectrum disorders. After all, failure to attribute feelings to a stuffed animal is perhaps an early sign of problems with theory of mind.

Ability to achieve "joint attention"

A really cool limousine passes by. The child excitedly points to it, so that you can share in the experience with him. This important form of social communication is called "joint attention"—you are jointly sharing the same experience. Note that the child isn't pointing simply to use you as a mechanical tool, such as pointing to the refrigerator so that you will satisfy his thirst for milk. Delayed ability to point for joint attention may be a marker for an ASD, even before delayed speech is noticed. After all, if you have theory of mind problems, with whom would you be sharing the experience?

Non-verbal (non-spoken) transmission of language

The simple sounds are not the only thing my body sends through space when it attempts to communicate with you. It also transmits:

- facial expressions—poor eye contact is a strong marker of ASD

- body language

- tone and prosody (rhythm) of speech.

Narrow and/or repetitive range of interests or behaviors

Rather than socializing, an autistic person has an inappropriately intense fascination with a particular subject, or may be overly preoccupied with the parts of an object. Typically, the child is inflexible and has ritualistic behaviors, including repetitive body movements such as rocking, spinning, or arm flapping. He may know every baseball statistic, or recognize any brand of car. Instead of carrying a stuffed animal around, he may perseverate on a rolled up piece of paper. This type of restricted or repetitive behavior is a major qualifying criterion for an ASD.

Secondary problems resulting from failure to understand

If the child does not understand what is going on around her—especially if pragmatic/socialization cues are difficult—secondary problems usually occur in ASDs. The child will frequently appear:

- *anxious*, since she doesn't know what she is supposed to do, or where the next blunder will come from

- *insistent on sameness* and show ritualistic behavior. Change means that previously hard-learned strategies will not help in this situation. These kids are barely hanging on. One new wrinkle can throw them over the edge. For example, Jill may know that her first task each day is to take her lunch out of the backpack. What happens, though, if today there is only half a day of school, and the lunch is missing? Now what does she do? The child may be unraveled for the rest of the day

- *concrete, and literal, and fail to see shades of grey*, for example, the child may have trouble with the concept of "white lies," because lies are bad, and that's the end of the story

- *inattentive*, since it's hard to pay attention to something she does not understand. The majority of children with an ASD also have ADHD

- *rude*, since she doesn't understand rules of conversation such as waiting your turn

- *interested in objects rather than people*; after all, objects are more predictable

- *to be "hanging back"* from peers, for all of the above reasons, and from simply not knowing how to make conversation and relate

- *"out of it"* and "odd" looking

- *socially unwelcome*. This can become quite painful, especially as the child gets older. Says Willey, "To choose to be left out is one thing, but to be locked out is quite another... I was crippled when I found out that it took more than I had to give to make new friends" (Willey 1999, p.72).

Categories of communication/socialization disorders: sorting them out

When a child has difficulties in these areas out of proportion to his general cognitive abilities, he can be considered to have a communication/socialization disorder.

Difficulties in the above skills can group together in varying combinations and severities, allowing for the naming of several communication disorder syndromes. As we shall see, these disorders overlap greatly. Some may even be duplicates of the same condition but approached by different specialties. Additionally, as children develop, their diagnostic classification might change. The human brain is not so simple that its disorders fit into neat, static categories. That is largely why DSM-5 uses the single umbrella term "Autism Spectrum Disorder" for what has been in the past a series of conditions under the umbrella "The Pervasive Developmental Disorders." Nonetheless, we present below the terminology of the last several decades, as many children carry these diagnoses, and the terms still prevail in research, school and diagnostic reports, and other texts. Furthermore, unless we still attempt to find certain patterns, and unless we know about the range of syndromes, we will fail to look for important symptoms that need to be addressed. More about the DSM-5 categorization of ASD is coming later.

Disorders of the communication skills are grouped into two major types of disorders. Let's give an overview of the organizational scheme first, and then come back to each condition in detail.

1. *Typical language-based learning disorders* are due to problems in the purely spoken/written language communication skills. These include expressive, receptive, processing, and articulation language disorders. Most routine speech and language evaluations examine these areas. Note that routine psychological testing (such as the WISC "IQ"—Wechsler Intelligence Scale for Children) examines areas of cognition (thinking), rather than language per se.

2. *Autism spectrum disorders (ASDs)* are those that include non-spoken communication/socialization problems—in particular, problems with back-and-forth socialization/ empathy. In other words, ASDs all share trouble with theory of mind, socialization, the pragmatics of language, and representational play. They may occur with or without additional verbal speech problems.

In turn, the autism spectrum disorders have been written about in two groupings:

- pervasive developmental disorders

- other autism spectrum disorders.

The *pervasive developmental disorders* (PDDs), defined medically in DSM-IV by the American Psychiatric Association, were a series of five diagnoses, of which autistic disorder is the most commonly discussed. "Pervasive" means that the problem cuts across multiple types of communication/socialization. Note that "PDD" is technically an overlying *category* (or "heading") for a group of actual individual specific diagnoses. So, it is better to talk of "the PDDs." These five PDDs are:

- *autistic disorder*—severely disordered verbal *and* non-verbal language; unusual or restrictive behaviors; commonly referred to as "autism"

- *Asperger's syndrome*—relatively good verbal language, with "milder" non-verbal language problems; restricted range of interests and relatedness

- *PDD-NOS* (not otherwise specified)—non-verbal language problems not meeting strict criteria for other PDD disorders

- *Rett's syndrome*—rare neurodegenerative disorder of girls

- *childhood disintegrative disorder*—a rare disorder that needs to be carefully distinguished from a neurodegenerative condition.

Meanwhile, the rest of the world has extended the spectrum beyond those conditions discussed in DSM-IV to include *other autistic spectrum disorders*. These terms have not been formally integrated into DSM-IV or DSM-5 vocabulary. Presumably, they were subsumed under the category of PDD-NOS in DSM-IV and are simply part of the Autism Spectrum Disorder category of DSM-5. In summary, these include:

- *high-functioning autism*—for some authors, this is synonymous with Asperger's; for others, it implies milder autism without retardation. It's perhaps better not to use this poorly defined term

- *non-verbal learning disabilities*—someone who has trouble integrating information in three areas: non-verbal difficulties causing the child to miss the major gestalt in language; spatial perception problems; and motor coordination problems

- *semantic-pragmatic language disorder*—delay and trouble with the use of language (both semantic and pragmatic), but socialization urge is relatively spared

- *hyperlexia*—most notable for incredible rote reading skills starting at an early age

- *some aspects of ADHD* (attention deficit hyperactivity disorder)—the impulsivity and self-control difficulties in ADHD may cause kids to have trouble showing their empathy.

DSM-IV pervasive developmental disorders

We start our more detailed review of each autistic spectrum disorder by presenting a summary of the key diagnostic criteria for each of the five PDD disorders as defined in DSM-IV (APA 1994).

Autistic disorder

By DSM-IV criteria, children with autistic disorder must have problems in each of the following three areas:

1. *Social interaction problems.* There are significant problems with non-verbal communication such as body language, eye contact, and facial expressions. Peer relationships are inadequate, and the child has trouble returning emotions during interactions. The person does not seek to share achievements or interests via pointing or bringing things for praise.

2. *Communication problems.* There are significant spoken language problems (which are not compensated for by signing). The person has trouble keeping up or starting a conversation (in those children who can speak). The speech tends to be stereotyped and/or repetitive. There is also a lack of communication via imaginative or imitative play.

3. *Narrow and/or repetitive range of interests or behaviors.* The autistic person has an inappropriately intense fascination with a particular subject, or may be overly preoccupied with the parts of an object. Typically, the child is inflexible and has ritualistic behaviors, including repetitive body movements such as rocking or arm flapping.

Other qualifying criteria include early onset (before three years old) of problems in at least one of the areas of: pretend/imaginary play, social interactions, or the pragmatic use of language.

Asperger's syndrome

The official DSM-IV criteria for Asperger's (APA 1994) are similar to those for autistic disorder, except they do not include the "communication" problem areas above. In other words, Asperger's people are autistic people who talk well. Although verbal speech is preserved in Asperger's, other communication problems certainly exist.

Symptoms of Asperger's include:

- impaired ability to utilize social cues such as body language or tone of voice
- impaired ability to understand irony or other "subtext" of communication
- "concrete" thinking
- restricted eye contact and socialization
- appearance as distant or a loner
- limited range of encyclopedic interests
- perseverative, odd behaviors
- over-sensitivity to certain stimuli
- unusual movements
- didactic, verbose, monotone, droning voice.

You can hear a soundtrack of two children with Asperger's at the author's website at www.pediatricneurology.com/aspergers_sound.htm. Once you hear their typical droning voice, you'll never forget it. It sounds as if the person is more interested in hearing the sound of his own speech than in communicating an idea to another person.

Asperger's syndrome is discussed in greater detail in the following chapter.

PDD-NOS (PDD-not otherwise specified)

The diagnosis of PDD-NOS is used for children on the autistic spectrum who do not completely fit into one of the other categories.

Rett's syndrome

This is a neurodegenerative disorder of girls who have normal initial development, but then show marked loss of developmental milestones and social interactions, slowing of head growth, and wringing hand movements.

Childhood disintegrative disorder

Children with this disorder develop normally for at least the first two years, and then have a deterioration sufficient to meet criteria for autistic disorder; but also show deterioration of language, muscle control, social, play, and toilet training skills. These children need to be carefully evaluated for an underlying neurodegenerative process.

Expanded autistic spectrum disorders

Next, we turn our attention to those autistic spectrum disorders that were not included in DSM-IV.

High-functioning autism

For some authors, this term is synonymous with Asperger's syndrome. For others, it implies milder autism without retardation, or PDD-NOS. Given the lack of consensus for the meaning of this term, it is probably best not to use it.

Non-verbal learning disabilities (NVLD or NLD)

Non-verbal learning disabilities (NVLDs) are a cluster of symptoms presumably related to poor ability to integrate information. These children have trouble with the ability to integrate it all together, i.e., to see the big gestalt picture rather than the details. In short, they "can't see the forest for the trees." These tasks are usually carried out by the brain's non-dominant hemisphere (typically the right hemisphere). Even though rote verbal language is spared, non-verbal areas of difficulty may be debilitating.

Although verbal communication is highly prized in school (good talkers, readers, and writers), up to two-thirds of communication actually occurs non-verbally (Thompson 1996). Thus, in the long run, the maladaptive learning of NVLD may be more destructive than typical LD. Estimates are that 0.1 to 1% of the population has an NVLD, compared with perhaps as much as 10% of the population having an LD (Thompson

1996), although these numbers may be an artifact of who and how we test.

Difficulty integrating non-verbal information occurs in three main areas:

1. *Motor skills:*

   - *Gross motor*—clumsy, unbalanced walking leading to clinging behaviors, bumping into things, fear of climbing, hesitant to explore physically, difficulty bike-riding, and uncoordinated at sports.

   - *Fine motor*—difficulty using scissors, shoe tying (which she'll talk herself through), and poor handwriting using awkward and tight grip.

2. *Visual/spatial orientation skills*, with an inability to form visual images.

   - Resultant focus on detail rather than the important gestalt.

   - Labels everything verbally, since that is the only— albeit not always accurate—way she can process the visual/spatial information. For example, she may find her way home by counting houses and labeling landmarks verbally.

   - The elaborate "naming" strategies break down with changes in routine, leading to an inability to cope with change.

   - Unaware where she is in space, unaware of where to place answers on the homework sheet, or how to navigate the school.

3. *Social/communication skills:*

   - Trouble integrating non-verbal communication with verbal communication in order to achieve full social interaction.

- Clearly appears to want social acceptance (versus Asperger's, where the children usually do not appear interested socially).

- Very literal interpretation of others; concrete thinking; seeing the world in black and white; trouble understanding dishonesty; trouble seeing hidden meanings, prompting others to say, "You know what I meant!"—when they didn't.

- Doesn't read the social cues of give-and-take conversation, thus appearing self-centered, weird, or impolite.

- Typically labeled as "annoying" because of their dependence on others, their constant speech, and their misinterpretation of social cues.

NVLD is determined by neuropsychological testing, whereas Asperger's is determined by detailed history and observation. There is great overlap in these two conditions—perhaps due to co-morbidity; or perhaps, as some authors feel, they are essentially the same condition but labeled by different specialties. However, people with Asperger's are primarily notable for *not appearing* interested in forming human bonds. (The degree to which Asperger's kids actually are painfully aware of their trouble making bonds is debated in the literature. Nevertheless, they typically appear uninterested.) NVLD kids, though, do typically appear interested in human bonds—even though they may be clueless about how to actually achieve them successfully. Additionally, children with Asperger's typically have more diminished "symbolic play" than children with NVLD. NVLD is not characterized by the repetitive or restricted range of interests that is required to meet Asperger's criteria.

So, how about this for a gross over-simplification? NVLD kids recognize that you exist, while they miss the subtext of what you are saying. Asperger's kids appear as if outside a window, as they miss the subtext of what you are saying.

Semantic-pragmatic language disorder (SPLD)

"Semantics" refers to the ability to use and understand words, phrases, and sentences, including abstract concepts and idioms. "Pragmatics" refers to the practical ability to use language in a social setting, such as knowing what is appropriate to say, where and when to say it, the give-and-take nature of a conversation, and the ability to know what the other person does or does not already know. Thus, semantic-pragmatic language disorder (SPLD) kids have:

- difficulty understanding the literal meaning of words and sentences (semantics)

- difficulty with abstract words, words about emotions, idioms, and words about status such as "expert" (semantics)

- difficulty extracting the central idea (pragmatics)

- trouble with the appropriate rules of conversation, such as talking "at" you or using monologues (pragmatics).

This inability to understand verbal language and the purpose of language leads to the typical secondary problems we have discussed above.

Here is what we might expect in the life of a child with SPLD through the years.

- They are often very easy infants.

- They may have delayed development of speech with few words even by two years old.

- They may have trouble with creative or symbolic play.

- Simple speech improves with therapy, but in school the child is "odd."

- They have good rote skills in math and computers, perhaps, but poor writing and socialization skills.

- They parrot back more than they understand, leading to an aura of intellectual maturity out of sync with their social skills.

- They have trouble understanding what others are really thinking or feeling, i.e., trouble with theory of mind.

- Many children with SPLD have fine motor problems; some also have gross motor difficulties.

- They may have trouble knowing what is socially acceptable, but are not usually conduct disorder teens.

- They may be "eccentric" adults.

SPLD can be differentiated from Asperger's in the following ways:

- SPLD kids tend to have more early speech delays than those with Asperger's.

- SPLD kids tend to have somewhat better socialization skills than those with Asperger's.

- The appropriate label may change over time as the child matures.

Hyperlexia

Hyperlexia is a condition, occurring almost always in boys, where autistic spectrum symptoms are accompanied by a striking capacity for rote reading. By 18–24 months of age, these kids have taught themselves the ability to name letters and numbers. By three years old, they may read printed words, exceeding even their ability to talk. By five years old, all have a fascination with the printed word. Some of the children seemed to have a mild regression at 18–24 months (less severe than as in autism).

In addition to this unusual reading skill, there are the other typical common autistic spectrum disorder symptoms we have seen.

Some aspects of ADHD

ADHDers typically have adequate capacity for empathy—but may have trouble inhibiting their behavior long enough to *show* it. Conversely, many children on the autistic spectrum may appear to have a short attention span, but this may actually be due to an inability to stay focused on situations they don't understand. Of course, ADHD and ASD can—and do—frequently co-occur as parts of the syndrome mix.

It is probably best to consider ADHD not as part of, but as sometimes sharing the following symptoms with autistic spectrum disorders:

- *Poor reading of social cues*—"Johnny, you're such a social klutz. Can't you see that the other children think that's weird?"

- *Poor ability to utilize "self-talk" to work through a problem*— "Johnny, what were you thinking?! Did you ever think this through?"

- *Poor sense of self-awareness*—Johnny's true answer to the above question is probably: "I don't have a clue. I guess I wasn't actually thinking."

- *Better performance with predictable routine.*

- *Poor generalization of rules*—"Johnny, I told you to shake hands with your teachers. Why didn't you shake hands with the *principal*?"

Summary of the past decades of terminology of ASDs

The classification of ASDs is in a state of flux. Since DSM-IV was published in 1994, a confusing and poorly defined "system" of terminology arose, with no single "official group" embracing or validating all of the categories. As we shall see shortly, the whole system has been tossed out in DSM-5. However, we have preserved the terms in this text since so many people still (and will continue to) carry these diagnostic groupings.

With trepidation, I offer the following gross over-simplifications of the terms used over the last several decades, and still in common use. I am reminded of my professor's comment on the first day of medical school, "One third of what I am going to tell you this year is wrong. Unfortunately, I don't know which third."

- ASDs are marked by difficulty in communication/socialization in areas other than the literal meaning of words (along with a restrictive/repetitive range of interests).

- Once a child has trouble with getting the big picture of communication and socialization, there will often be secondary symptoms, such as anxiety, holding back from peers, a rigid adherence to sameness, a relative preference for things (which are predictable) rather than people, and an appearance of "oddness."

- Asperger's and autism share primarily the difficulty of recognizing the existence of others—trouble with theory of mind. People with Asperger's can talk; autism usually has limited speech.

- Asperger's children *appear* less interested in forming bonds and have more trouble with "theory of mind" than NVLD and semantic-pragmatic language disorder.

- NVLDs are marked by integration problems of pragmatic language gestalt, spatial orientation, and motor coordination.

- Hyperlexia is marked by fascination with the printed word starting at an early age.

- "High-functioning autism" is used by different authors to mean autistic disorder with relatively spared speech and cognition, Asperger's syndrome, or PDD-NOS.

Autistic spectrum disorders such as Asperger's tend to be highly "co-morbid"—they occur in conjunction with other conditions of the syndrome mix. ADHD, anxiety, obsessive-compulsive disorder (OCD), and sensory integration problems are particularly common.

DSM-5 and ASD

The old criteria of DSM-IV just weren't working out. Most importantly, scientific consensus has reached the conclusion that all of the different DSM-IV PDD disorders (except Rett's syndrome, which never should have been put in a psychiatric classification, anyway) were all manifestations of a single disorder with varying degrees of severity in the areas of social communication and restricted/repetitive behaviors. Thus, in DSM-5, all of the variants discussed above have been placed into a single condition entitled "Autism Spectrum Disorder."

DSM-5 criteria for ASD

Two basic criteria need to be fulfilled in the new DSM-5 criteria for ASD: problems in the area of social communication; and problems with repetitive, narrow, restricted, or odd behaviors or interests.

1. *Problems with social interaction and social communication* are delineated into three closely related areas, simplified as follows.

   a. *Problems with social and emotional reciprocity*, i.e., the ability, "to engage with others and share thoughts and feelings" in a back-and-forth fashion (APA 2013, p.53).

   b. *Problems with the non-verbal communication skills* required for the ability to carry out those social interactions. These diminished skills include body language, eye contact, and other non-verbal skills (such as comprehending subtext or hidden messages).

   c. *Problems with understanding, forming, and sustaining relationships*, ranging from trouble figuring out how to act in different social settings, to shared pretend play, to lack of urge to form bonds.

2. *Narrow, repetitive range of interests or behaviors* (at least two of the following):

   a. *Stereotypical or repeated behaviors*, such as flapping, use of repetitive phrases, echoing back what was just said, or lining up objects.

   b. *Inflexible need for sameness or routine*, such as becoming unraveled if the bus takes a different route to school today.

   c. *Unusually deep fascination with topics or objects*, such as memorizing the New York City subway map, or knowing everything about insects, or fixation with unusual objects, such as carrying around a spoon.

   d. *Increased and/or decreased sensitivity to stimuli*, such as fascination with spinning objects, sniffing objects, or avoidance/seeking of certain tastes or textures or other sensations. (This sounds awfully like sensory integration dysfunction. See Chapter 8.)

Once again, there are the usual qualifiers: the symptoms must begin (although not necessarily be recognized) in early childhood, must interfere with the quality of life, and must not be better explained by something else.

Although many people have been distressed that DSM-5 lumps everything together under the single ASD umbrella, it actually allows a number of "specifiers" that indeed allow for a better description of an individual on the spectrum—certainly better than the old non-specific term PDD-NOS. These include specifiers as follows:

- *Each of the two main categories above—social communication and restricted/repetitive behaviors—are each rated independently as either: Level 1 ("requiring support"), Level 2 ("requiring substantial support"), or Level 3 ("requiring very substantial support").* Note that "the descriptive severity categories should not be used to determine eligibility for and provision of services; these can only be developed at an individual level and through discussion of personal priorities and targets" (APA 2013, p.51).

- *With or without accompanying intellectual impairment* (give brief description of level).

- *With or without accompanying language impairment* (give brief description of level).

- *Specify if an associated neurobehavioral disorder exists* (such as ADHD, Tourette's, etc.).

- *Specify if associated with a known medical/genetic condition* (such as Rett's syndrome or epilepsy).

See Chapter 6 for additional discussion of DSM-5 naming conventions regarding the ASDs—particularly regarding Asperger's syndrome.

Social (pragmatic) communication disorder

To meet DSM-5 criteria for autism communication disorder, a child must meet both criteria above of social communication and restricted/repetitive behaviors. If the person meets criteria for the socialization criteria above, but there is no evidence (now or from past history) of the narrow/repetitive criteria, then the correct diagnosis would probably be the newly created "Social (Pragmatic) Communication Disorder."

Simplified criteria from DSM-5 include all of the following problems in the social use of verbal and non-verbal communication.

- Using communication for social ends.

- Matching communication style to the needs of the listener (e.g., speaking differently to a child versus an adult).

- Following the rules of give-and-take conversation and of narrating a story.

- Deducing what isn't explicitly said, such as inference and subtext.

Importantly, note that this social (pragmatic) communication disorder does not even mention trouble with the *urge* to socialize. In fact, DSM-5 places this disorder under the heading of "Communication Disorders" and is not in the ASD section. These are the kids who have the urge, but not the ability, to fit in socially (and, to repeat, never had the problem with restricted/ repetitive behaviors). The condition is not usually diagnosable until the child is four to five years of age, but may not be apparent until early adolescence.

Notice that DSM-5 now actually makes clear that "communication" is a means to the end of "socialization" in both ASD and social communication disorder.

Treatment of ASD

The treatment of the less severe form of ASD is discussed in depth in Dr. Attwood's following chapter. More severely affected children require more intensive treatment. General rules of intensive treatment include the following (Myers 2007):

- Start as early as the diagnosis is seriously considered.

- Carry out the treatment for 25 hours per week for 12 months/year.

- The treatment should be of long duration (years).

- It should utilize a great deal of 1:1 attention.

- It should include a parent training component.

- It should utilize close, specific monitoring of progress.

These principles apply to such programs as Applied Behavioral Analysis (ABA), where the rewards that motivate the child are analyzed and then applied in discrete educational trials to teach one small behavior or skill after another. A recent meta-analysis of the literature of ABA programs found a dose-related response on both language and adaptive skills with respect to hours/week and duration in months or years (Maglione *et al.* 2012), i.e., the more, the better. Further information on these treatments can be found at www.nationalautismcenter.org/learning/parent_manual.php or in the Further Reading section of this book.

Also, we must be sure to look for other associated conditions of the syndrome mix, as around 70% of people on the autism spectrum have one other mental disorder, and 40% have two or more (APA 2013, p.58). Precautions against a spectrum child's wandering or running away (with all of the risks including drowning) can be found at www.awaare.org. See Chapter 14 for information on medical and complementary treatments.

CHAPTER 6

Autism Spectrum Disorder, Level 1 (Asperger's Syndrome) and its Treatment

Tony Attwood, PhD

Children who have an Autism Spectrum Disorder have discovered activities more interesting and enjoyable than socializing. Unfortunately, their peers are social zealots.

The previous chapter has explained the new diagnostic criteria for an Autism Spectrum Disorder (ASD) in the recent *Diagnostic and Statistical Manual of Mental Disorders* (DSM-5) published by the American Psychiatric Association (2013). The DSM-5 guidelines recommend that the multi-disciplinary team conducting the diagnostic assessment also describes any associated developmental disabilities, medical and psychiatric factors, and level of expression. The term *specifiers* has been created to describe additional information relevant to the diagnosis, in particular:

- with or without accompanying intellectual impairment

- with or without accompanying language impairment

- association with a known medical or genetic condition or environmental factor

- association with another neurodevelopmental, mental or behavior disorder, or catatonia

- severity of expression from Level 1 to Level 3 based on the level of support needed for social communication and for restricted, repetitive behaviors. The DSM-5 text clearly states that the level of severity should not be used to determine eligibility for and provision of services, as these can only be developed at an individual level and through discussion of personal priorities and targets.

Although the field has not yet settled on the exact wording, an example of the diagnostic profile for an ASD using the new *specifiers* would be:

> James is a teenager who has an ASD at Level 1 for both social communication and restricted, repetitive behaviors, without language or intellectual impairment, and in association with Attention Deficit Hyperactivity Disorder and Generalized Anxiety Disorder.

Asperger's syndrome

A separate diagnostic category of Asperger's Disorder or Asperger's syndrome is not included in the DSM-5, but clinicians, therapists, teachers, parents, and those with an ASD Level 1 ("requires services") can still use the term Asperger's syndrome, which has been in general usage for over two decades. The concept of Asperger's syndrome has not suddenly disappeared; it will be replaced with the new diagnostic term *ASD Level 1* and relevant specifiers. According to the authors of DSM-5, all children and adults who had a previous diagnosis of Asperger's syndrome or PDD-NOS should be given the diagnosis of ASD.

In my own clinical practice, I use the new DSM-5 diagnostic criteria and state that a child has *ASD Level 1 without language or intellectual impairment (Asperger's syndrome)* so that parents, teachers, and therapists will be able to use a term, namely Asperger's syndrome, that is often understood by the general public. Asperger's syndrome is also a term that can be used to seek further information from the internet and published books, and research articles published prior to 2013. Thus, the term will still be legitimately used by clinicians, parents, teachers, therapists, and those with an ASD. The general public will also continue to use the term in conversations, and the media will also probably continue to use the term Asperger's syndrome rather than ASD Level 1.

My personal opinion is that the new DSM-5 criteria are an improvement on the old criteria and consistent with advances in clinical wisdom and academic research. Although I will lament the removal of the term Asperger's syndrome from the DSM, I agree with the rationale and know that the term will remain in common usage.

Catatonia

One of the specifiers for ASD is catatonia. During adolescence, a teenager, or young adult who has an ASD may have a marked deterioration in movement abilities, with a slowing and "freezing" of movement mid-action, and symptoms of mutism, posturing, grimacing, and waxy flexibility. Should a deterioration in movement abilities occur, an assessment is warranted by a specialist in the movement disorders associated with ASD.

Stricter diagnostic criteria

DSM-5 uses stricter diagnostic criteria than DSM-IV and this will have an impact on the future number of children diagnosed with an ASD. It is too early to tell in 2013, when this chapter is being written, how the diagnostic landscape will change, but it appears that there may be a future decrease in the number of children achieving a diagnosis of ASD.

For simplicity, this chapter will use the brief two-word term "Asperger's syndrome" rather than the new nine-word diagnostic term "Autism Spectrum Disorder Level 1 without language or intellectual impairment."

Are there any gender differences?

Girls who have Asperger's syndrome are primarily different to the boys—not regarding the core characteristics of ASD, but rather in their reaction to being different. Girls often use more constructive coping and adjustment strategies to effectively camouflage their confusion in social situations and may achieve superficial social success by imitating others or avoiding engagement in interpersonal situations until they have learned what to do to achieve successful social inclusion.

A girl with Asperger's syndrome can become an avid observer of other children and intellectually determine what to do in social situations: she learns to imitate other girls, adopts an alternative persona, and acts as someone who can succeed in social situations. In effect, she becomes a social chameleon. On the other hand, some girls escape into a world of imagination. They constructively avoid social interactions with other children, choosing instead to engage in creative solitary play, read fiction, or spend time with animals.

Girls with Asperger's syndrome often prefer to play with typical boys, whose play is more constructive and adventurous than emotional and conversational. Many women who have Asperger's syndrome have described to psychologists and in autobiographies how they sometimes think they have a male rather than a female brain, having a greater understanding and appreciation of the interests, thinking, and humor of boys during their early school years. The girl may be described as a tomboy, eager to join in the activities and conversations of boys rather than those of girls, and she develops talents in school subjects that are predominantly male dominated, such as mathematics and science. The girl with Asperger's syndrome may not follow society's expectations of femininity. For example, she may prefer to wear practical, comfortable, "masculine" clothing rather than dressing in a fashionable or feminine way. During adolescence, she may also have an aversion for the tactile and sensory aspects of makeup and perfume. During their adolescence, some girls with Asperger's syndrome use the strategy of being extremely well behaved and compliant in class so as not to be noticed or recognized as different by the teacher; they are often known at school for their exemplary good behavior.

Adolescent girls with Asperger's syndrome are often late to develop romantic relationships, having an almost puritanical attitude towards intimacy. Their first intimate experiences can be several years later than peers. There is an alternative trajectory: adolescent girls with Asperger's syndrome can develop low self-esteem due to bullying and teasing by peers, and rather than follow social and moral conventions, decide to actively contradict them, becoming vulnerable at a relatively early age to relationships and even to sexual predation. They may not have the intuitive ability to identify disreputable characters, tend to set their relationship expectations very low, and often experience multiple abusive relationships.

These coping and camouflaging mechanisms, and having friendships with boys rather than girls, often mask the characteristics of Asperger's syndrome during the elementary school years. However, there is a psychological cost that may become apparent only in adolescence. It is emotionally exhausting to be constantly observing and analyzing the social behavior of other girls, and trying not to make a social error. Adopting an alternative persona can lead to confusion with self-identity and low self-esteem. The stress, strain, and exhaustion of intellectually analyzing social situations and acting "normal" with female peers but still being rejected, bullied, and teased can result in the development of depression, an anxiety disorder, eating disorder, or borderline personality disorder. The clinician diagnosing or treating these secondary mood or personality disorders may then identify the characteristics of Asperger's syndrome when exploring the developmental history of the girl. Psychologists and psychiatrists therefore need a paradigm shift in their recognition of the female presentation of Asperger's syndrome to ensure earlier diagnosis and access to effective understanding and support for girls with Asperger's syndrome.

Adjustment to being different

By definition, a child with a developmental disorder such as Asperger's syndrome is different from other children. However, the child with Asperger's syndrome will have also recognized that he or she is different from other children. Some children with Asperger's syndrome will internalize their emotional reaction to being different, while others externalize their emotional reaction.

Internalizing thoughts and feelings
Depression

Children with Asperger's syndrome do not know intuitively how to play or interact with their peers, and can be subject to ridicule, teasing, and rejection—leading to damaged self-esteem. Social competence and friendship abilities are highly valued by typical children, and not being successful in these abilities can lead some children with Asperger's syndrome to internalize their thoughts and feelings with self-criticism, increased social withdrawal, and feelings of being defective. Such children, sometimes as young as six years, may then develop a reactive depression as a result of insight into being different. From my clinical experience of treating depression in teenagers who have Asperger's syndrome, many have internalized the derogatory comments of peers and believe they are a loser, stupid, or "psycho," and perceive their experiences as confirming those beliefs.

Imagination

A more constructive internalization of thoughts and feelings of being different can be to escape into imagination. The child develops a vivid and complex alternative world in terms of periods of history, such as the time of dinosaurs (no people or school), or ancient Egypt (life was simpler), or a future world based on technology, such as science fiction films. Sometimes the loneliness can lead to the creation of imaginary friends, who are the friends the child would like to have.

In this imaginary or fantasy world, the child is successful and respected. The degree of imaginative thought and frequent practice can lead to an avid interest in reading and writing fiction. The escape into imagination can be a psychologically constructive adaptation, but there are risks during adolescence, when this retreat into a fantasy world may lead to the exclusion of other activities, and to other people misinterpreting the adolescent's intentions or state of mind. The intense enjoyment of being in an imaginary world may also be a stark contrast to the boring world of the classroom and the vulnerable world of the playground. The child may then be viewed as inattentive, distracted and "in a world of his own."

Externalizing thoughts and feelings
Anger and arrogance

An alternative to internalizing negative thoughts and feelings about being different is to externalize them, "It is not my fault, but your fault." The child may over-compensate for the lack of competence in social situations by completely denying any problems and developing a sense of superiority and anger towards others, and an inflated or narcissistic self-esteem. Suggestions from remedial programs or therapy are vehemently rejected. The child can also become arrogant, which may lead to conduct problems. Unfortunately, one of the consequences of arrogance, denial, and the immaturity of appreciating the thoughts, intentions, and perspectives of others, is to seek resolution and retribution for social embarrassment by physical retaliation.

Imitation

A more psychologically constructive way of externalizing thoughts and feelings of being different is to observe and imitate the characteristics of those peers who are socially successful. The child learns from intense observation of peers how to "act" in social situations. Some children with Asperger's syndrome, especially girls, can be remarkably astute in their observation abilities, copying gestures, tone of voice, mannerisms, and style of dress. This can be a constructive way of achieving social inclusion as long as the child mimics an appropriate role model.

Unfortunately, some adolescents with Asperger's syndrome may imitate the socially popular but notorious "bad guys" at school, which leads to concerns regarding behavior and morality. The presentation of a false self, "faking it till you make it," and wearing a "mask" to hide the inner self can be successful but exhausting, and can contribute to having low self-esteem, and the real self must remain secret. This strategy for coping with being different can also contribute to depression in the adult years.

Should you explain the diagnosis to the child?

The answer is a resounding "yes." Clinical experience indicates that explaining the diagnosis to the child with Asperger's syndrome is extremely important. This will help prevent the development of inappropriate compensatory mechanisms, and encourage the child to accept treatment programs.

When I conduct a diagnostic assessment of ASD in adults, I often ask, "When would you have wanted to know exactly why you were different and that you have Asperger's syndrome?" The overwhelming response is, "As young as possible, then I wouldn't have felt so stupid or defective, people would have understood and helped me, and I could have accessed specialists to teach me the skills I needed."

The Attributes Activity

In the Attributes Activity that I have developed and use clinically is a listing of the child's "Qualities" (i.e., "Strengths") and "Difficulties," which helps to explain the diagnosis to the child and his or her family. The clinician gathers close family members, including the person who has recently been diagnosed as having Asperger's syndrome. First, large sheets of paper are attached to the wall, or a large whiteboard with colored pens can be used. Each sheet is divided into two columns: "Qualities (Strengths)" and "Difficulties."

I usually suggest that another family member, mother, or father, is the first person to complete the activity, which is to identify his or her own personal qualities and difficulties. These can include practical abilities, knowledge, personality, and the expression and management of feelings. After the initial focus person has made some suggestions, which the clinician writes on the paper/board, the family members add their own suggestions. The clinician ensures that this is a positive activity, commenting on the various attributes and ensuring there are more qualities/ strengths than difficulties. The child with Asperger's syndrome is then able to observe and participate in the activity, and understand what is expected when it is his or her turn.

The clinician comments on each quality and difficulty nominated by the child with Asperger's syndrome and then explains that scientists are often looking for patterns and theories. When they find a consistent pattern, they like to give it a name after the first person to identify that pattern or theory, such as Einstein's Theory of Relativity or Newton's Theory of Gravity. Reference is then made to Dr. Hans Asperger who, over 70 years ago, saw at his clinic in Vienna many children with a pattern of similar characteristics of qualities and difficulties as the child who is completing this activity. He published the first clinical description of this pattern that has become known as Asperger's syndrome.

I usually say to the child, "Congratulations, you have Asperger's syndrome," and explain that this means they are not mad, bad, or defective, but have a *different* way of thinking. The discussion continues with an explanation of how some of the child's talents or qualities are due to having Asperger's syndrome, such as impressing people with his or her knowledge about the Titanic, ability to draw with photographic realism, or to sing in perfect pitch, attention to detail, sensory sensitivity, and natural talent in mathematics, information technology, and engineering. This is to introduce to the child the benefits of having the characteristics of Asperger's syndrome.

Prior to adolescence, children who have a confirmed and explained diagnosis tend to be very positive with regard to peers knowing of the diagnostic label. However, this is often not the case with teenagers. Adolescents who have Asperger's syndrome are vulnerable to being bullied and teased, and are acutely aware that packs of adolescent "predators" are seeking someone who is labeled as different to become a target. Teenagers with Asperger's syndrome are usually very keen to be inconspicuous, having observed peers who have been singled out for bullying because of being different in terms of abilities, physique, or a psychiatric diagnosis. This can lead to a rejection of the diagnosis, not necessarily because of disagreement with the actual diagnosis, but fear of the diagnosis being used by peers for ridicule and rejection. Thus, it may be important that the diagnosis for adolescents is viewed as extremely confidential information and not disclosed to peers.

The next stage in the diagnostic assessment is to discuss the difficulties and the strategies needed to improve specific abilities at home and at school. This can include the advantages of guidance and counseling in social understanding, cognitive behavioral therapy or medication that is used to help with emotion management, and ideas to help with making friends and to cope with bullying and teasing. The clinician provides a summary of the person's qualities and difficulties that are due to having Asperger's syndrome and mentions successful people in the areas of science, information technology, politics, and the arts who benefited from the signs of Asperger's syndrome in their own profile of abilities—such as Einstein, Thomas Jefferson, and Mozart.

The activity closes with explanation of some of my personal thoughts on Asperger's syndrome. Such individuals have a different perception of the world, way of thinking, and set of priorities. The brain is wired differently not defectively. The person prioritizes the pursuit of knowledge, perfection, and truth, and the understanding of the physical world above feelings and interpersonal experiences. This can lead to valued talents, but also vulnerabilities in the social world of school. But consider this: Asperger's syndrome may be the next stage of human evolution.

Treatment programs
Making friends
The five stages of making friends

Having observed the social development of children, adolescents, and adults with Asperger's syndrome, I have identified five stages in the motivation and experience of friendships and relationships.

1. An interest in the physical world.

2. Wanting to play with friends.

3. Making friends.

4. Searching for a partner.

5. Maintaining the partnership.

1. AN INTEREST IN THE PHYSICAL WORLD

Very young children with Asperger's syndrome may not be interested in the activities of their peers. They are usually more interested in understanding the physical world than the social world, and may enter the preschool playground to explore the drainage system of the school or to search for insects and reptiles. The social activities of their peers are perceived as boring with incomprehensible social rules. The child is content with solitude; he or she is alone, not lonely.

2. WANTING TO PLAY WITH FRIENDS

In the early elementary school years, children with Asperger's syndrome recognize that other children are having fun socializing. They want to experience that enjoyment, and try to be included in the social activities of their peers. However, despite intellectual ability within the normal range, their level of social maturity is usually at least two years behind their peers, and they often have considerable difficulties with reciprocal and cooperative play. The child with Asperger's syndrome may long for social inclusion, social success, and a friend. This is the time when the child becomes acutely aware of being different to his or her peers and the adjustment strategies described above may begin.

3. MAKING FRIENDS

In the middle school years, the child may make genuine friendships. Friendships may be brief, with a tendency for the child with Asperger's syndrome to be too dominant or to have too rigid a view of friendship. Some typical children who are naturally kind, understanding, and "maternal" can be tolerant and become genuine friends. Sometimes the friendship is with similar, socially isolated children who share the same interests and diagnostic characteristics.

4. SEARCHING FOR A PARTNER

In late adolescence, teenagers with Asperger's syndrome may seek more than a superficial or platonic friendship with like-minded individuals and express a longing for a partner. They can be confused by the new, more complex, dimensions to adolescent friendships, especially aspects of self-disclosure, the communication of inner thoughts and feelings, romantic relationships, and sexuality. Adolescents with Asperger's syndrome often become more acutely aware that they are different from their peers. They may begin to seek a romantic partner rather than a friend; someone they believe will understand them and provide emotional support and guidance in the social world.

5. MAINTAINING THE PARTNERSHIP

Eventually, perhaps when emotionally and socially more mature, the adult with Asperger's syndrome may find a lifetime partner. However, both partners probably need relationship counseling to facilitate the adjustments needed in the relationship. We now have literature and relationship counseling programs specifically for couples where one partner has Asperger's syndrome.

Programs to encourage friendship skills

We now have therapy programs to encourage friendship skills in children and adolescents who have Asperger's syndrome. Parents may provide some guidance at home, but schools will need to be aware that they must develop a social curriculum for a child with

Asperger's syndrome with an emphasis on friendship skills, and provide appropriate teacher training and resources. The following treatment suggestions are designed for each of the developmental stages of friendship that occur in typical children.

Ages three to six years

AN ADULT ACTING AS A FRIEND

Very young children with Asperger's syndrome may prefer to interact and play with adults more than with peers. It is important that adults, especially parents, observe the natural play of the child's peers—noting the games, equipment, rules, and language. They can then practice the same play with the child but with an adult "acting" as his or her same-age friend. This includes using "child speak": namely, the speech of children rather than adults. It is important that the adult role-plays examples of being a good friend and also role-plays unfriendly acts, such as disagreements and teasing. Appropriate and inappropriate responses can be enacted to provide the child with a range of responses. Once the child has rehearsed with an adult, who can easily modify the pace of play and amount of instruction, he or she can practice social play with another child. Perhaps an older sibling can act as a friend, and provide further practice before the skills are used openly with the peer group.

In the early childhood years, a good friend is someone who shares, takes turns, and helps. It is important that when an adult is playing with the child, the activities involve an equivalent level of abilities and contribution in the choice of activity. Activities can be undertaken in a cooperative rather than competitive way. Turn taking should be a key feature of interactive play. For example, practice taking turns in finding and connecting each piece of a jigsaw puzzle. To encourage assistance, the adult can feign difficulty and ask the child for help, commenting that good friends help each other.

Barclay Public Library
220 South Main Street
PO Box 349
Warrensburg, IL 62573

SOCIAL DOCUMENTARIES

Use a video camera to make short and interesting videos of the child's everyday social experiences. For example, film the child playing with his or her peers in the sandpit, or involved in social games such as chasing, or hide-and-seek. The pause and replay buttons can be used to focus on particular cues and responses. Young children with Asperger's syndrome often enjoy watching videos and television. This activity can be used to improve friendship skills.

Ages six to nine years

At this stage, typical children start to recognize that they need a friend to play certain games, and that the friend must like those games. They become more aware of the thoughts and feelings of their peers and how their actions and comments can hurt both physically and emotionally. Most children are prepared sometimes to inhibit their intentions and to accept and incorporate the influences, preferences, and goals of their friends in their play. There is less of a dominant/submissive quality. Rather, helping—especially mutual help—is one of the indicators of friendship at this stage. Around the age of eight years, typical children develop the concept of a best friend as not only their first choice for social play, but also as someone who helps in practical terms: "She knows how to fix the computer," or "He cheers me up when I'm feeling sad."

SOCIAL STORIES™

Teacher and internationally recognized expert on children with ASD, Carol Gray, has developed the strategy of Social Stories™, which is remarkably effective in enabling the child to understand the cues and responses for specific social situations. The guidance is not only in what to do, but more importantly, why there are certain codes of social conduct and expectations. Children with Asperger's syndrome will need this type of practical guidance in relating to their peers in the playground and the classroom. A Social Story™ is written as a collaborative exercise between the adult and child, and the story is consistent with the child's reading ability. The Social Story™ describes a situation, skill, or concept in terms of relevant social cues, perspectives, and common responses. The goal is to share accurate social and emotional information in a reassuring and informative manner that is easily understood by the child with Asperger's syndrome. The first Social Story™ and at least 50 percent of subsequent Social Stories™ should describe, affirm, and consolidate existing abilities and knowledge, and what the child does well. This can avoid the problem of a Social Story™ being only associated with failure. Social Stories™ can also be written as a means of recording achievements in the use of new knowledge and strategies. Preparing Social Stories™ also enables others to understand the perspective of the child, and why his or her social behavior can appear unduly confused, anxious, aggressive, or disobedient.

Social Stories™ use positive language and a constructive approach. The suggestions are what to do rather than what not to do. The text will include *descriptive sentences* that provide factual information or statements; but one of the reasons for the success of Social Stories™ is the use of *perspective sentences*. These sentences are written to explain a person's perception of the mental world, and describe thoughts, emotions, beliefs, opinions, motivation, and knowledge. They are specifically included to improve theory of mind abilities. Carol Gray recommends including *cooperative sentences* to identify who can be of assistance, which can be a very important aspect of social assistance and emotion management, and *directive sentences* that suggest a response or choice of responses in a particular situation. *Affirmative sentences* explain a commonly shared value, opinion, or rule—the reason why specific codes of conduct have been established and why there is the expectation of conformity. *Control sentences* are written by the child to identify personal strategies to help remember what to do. The Social Story™ will also need a title, which should reflect its essential characteristics or criteria. Carol Gray has developed a Social Story™ formula such that the text describes more than directs. (See the Further Reading section for useful resources on Social Stories™.)

While a Social Story™ provides the rationale and script of what to do, there will also need to be opportunities to rehearse and practice new social understanding in real-life situations. Teachers and parents may rehearse aspects of social play with a small group of selected children who understand the difficulties of the child with Asperger's syndrome—a "dress rehearsal" before engaging in independent social play.

Ages 9 to 13 years

In the third stage of friendship, a friend is chosen because of special attributes in their abilities and personality. A friend is someone who genuinely cares, with complimentary attitudes, ideas, and values. There is a strong need to be liked and respected by one's peers, with a mutual sharing of experiences and thoughts. With increased self-disclosure, there is the recognition of being trustworthy and seeking advice not only for practical problems but also for interpersonal issues, and the need for a more constructive approach when disagreements occur. There is also a need for companionship and greater selectivity and durability in the friendship alliances. At this stage, there is a distinct gender split, and peer pressure becomes increasingly important. Peer group acceptance and values become more important than the opinion of parents. Friends also support each other in terms of managing emotions. If the child is sad, close friends can provide the necessary reassurance and optimism; if angry, they can provide the calm required to prevent him or her getting into trouble.

SOCIAL ENGINEERING

As the peer group becomes more important in establishing self-esteem, teachers and parents will need to undertake some "social engineering" with regard to how they group the children. Parents can identify a prospective friend and arrange a family outing or activity at home that includes the potential friend, with some careful monitoring and guidance to encourage an enjoyable time for both parties. They may need to encourage the peer group to consider the perspective of the child with Asperger's syndrome.

ENCOURAGING A BUDDY

Individual children who have a natural rapport with a child with Asperger's syndrome can be guided and encouraged to be a mentor in the classroom and playground, and in social situations. Their advice may be accepted as having greater value than that of parents or teachers. It is also important to encourage friends or peers to help children with Asperger's syndrome regulate their moods. Peers can step in and help them calm down if they are becoming agitated or tormented. Friends may need to provide reassurance if such children are anxious, and to cheer them up when sad. Children with Asperger's syndrome will also need advice and encouragement to give reciprocal emotional support. They will need to be taught how to recognize the signs of distress or agitation in their friends, and how to respond. Social Stories™ can be used for this age group, with the topics being aspects of friendship such as giving compliments, emotional support, and being a good listener.

TEAMWORK SKILLS

At this stage, some remedial programs use strategies to develop teamwork rather than friendship skills. Attending a program on teamwork skills for sports or employment may be considered more acceptable to young teenagers with Asperger's syndrome, who may be sensitive to any suggestion that they need remedial programs to have friends, or that they do not have friends.

INTERACTIVE COMPUTER GAMES

There are interactive computer games to teach social skills and emotional understanding specifically for children with Asperger's syndrome. The Secret Agent Society, developed in Queensland, Australia, has been specifically designed and evaluated for 8–12-year-olds who have Asperger's syndrome (see Further Reading section).

DRAMA CLASSES

Another strategy to help the young adolescent who is sensitive to being publicly identified as having few friends is to adapt speech and drama classes. This is an appropriate and effective strategy, especially for young teenagers. Those with Asperger's syndrome can learn and practice conversational scripts, self-disclosure, body language, facial expression, and tone of voice for particular situations, and role-play people they know who are socially successful, or role-play strategies to constructively manage being bullied, teased, or rejected.

Ages 13 to 18 years

In the previous developmental stage of friendship there may be a small core of close friends, but in this stage, the breadth and depth of friendship increases. There can be different friends for different needs, such as comfort, humor, or practical advice. A friend is defined as someone who, "accepts me for who I am" or "thinks the same way about things." A friend provides a sense of personal identity and is compatible with one's own personality.

SELF-HELP GUIDES

There are multiple sources of guidance. There are now several books published by Jessica Kingsley Publishers that have been written by teenagers with Asperger's syndrome as self-help guides for fellow teenagers.

SUPPORT GROUPS

This writer (Tony Attwood) has developed the concept of an Emotional Toolbox, a successful strategy for "cognitive restructuring"—one of the main activities used to help restructure or repair a specific feeling.

Parent support groups have also established regular meetings for adolescents with Asperger's syndrome to enable discussion of issues such as friendships, sexuality, and being bullied or rejected by peers. A team of parents usually coordinates the groups with advice from professionals who are often invited to the meetings and facilitate discussion and suggestions.

THE INTERNET

The internet has become the modern equivalent of the dance hall in terms of an opportunity for young people to meet. The great advantage of internet communication to people with Asperger's syndrome is that they often have a greater eloquence in disclosing and expressing their inner self and feelings through typing rather than conversation. However, parents will need to carefully supervise internet friendships, as teenagers with Asperger's syndrome are vulnerable to abuse from someone who appears to have friendly intentions.

Therapy suggestions for all stages in friendship

POSITIVE FEEDBACK

If completing a mathematics activity, children know they have the correct solution by confirming the answer on a calculator. When completing a jigsaw puzzle, they know they have been successful when all the pieces fit together and complete the picture. But how does a child with Asperger's syndrome know when he or she was "correct" in socializing? It is essential that adults and peers recognize, and comment on, what the child with Asperger's syndrome did in an interaction that was socially appropriate. Otherwise, the only feedback is criticism when he or she has made a social error. Children with Asperger's syndrome need more positive feedback than they typically receive when playing or socializing with peers.

BOOKS ON FRIENDSHIP

There are storybooks, novels, and guides written for typical children of various ages that describe and explore aspects of friendship. These books can be read to the child with Asperger's syndrome by parents, or chosen as class reading material and be the basis of class discussions.

THE ART OF CONVERSATION

Speech pathologists can provide individual and group activities to encourage the pragmatic aspects of language, that is, the use of language skills in a social context. Throughout all the stages of friendship, the child will need guidance in the pragmatic aspects of communication, including the "art of conversation," attentive listening, narrative abilities, and reading cues that indicate interest, boredom, or signal the end of the conversation.

PROGRAMS TO AVOID BEING TEASED AND BULLIED
The school may need to implement an anti-bullying program that can be modified for children with Asperger's syndrome. While we hope that social inclusion is a positive experience, inevitably the child with Asperger's syndrome will be the target for teasing, bullying, ridicule, and deliberate exclusion. We now have several specially designed programs to reduce the frequency and different types of bullying and teasing of children with Asperger's syndrome.

Managing emotions

Cognitive behavioral therapy

Research studies, clinical experience, and autobiographies have confirmed that children with Asperger's syndrome have considerable difficulty with the understanding and expression of emotions, and are at risk of developing an anxiety disorder, depression, or problems with anger management. Cognitive behavioral therapy (CBT) has been developed and refined by psychologists over several decades and, using rigorous scientific evaluations, proven to be effective in changing the way a typical person thinks about and responds to feelings such as anxiety, sadness, and anger. CBT focuses on aspects of direct applicability to children with Asperger's syndrome, who are known to have deficits and distortions in thinking about thoughts and feelings. We are now able to modify conventional CBT, which was designed for typical children, to accommodate the profile of abilities and experiences of children and adolescents with Asperger's syndrome, with increasingly positive results.

Affective education

CBT programs for children with Asperger's syndrome have two stages. The first stage is *affective education*, where the child learns about emotions. Children and adults who have Asperger's syndrome can have *Alexithymia*, that is, considerable difficulty identifying the specific word that describes a particular feeling. They also have considerable difficulty reading the non-verbal expressions of emotions in a person's face, tone of voice, and the social context. There can also be difficulty expressing complex or subtle emotions in *their own* facial expressions, body language, and speech. Thus, children and adolescents who have Asperger's syndrome need to improve their range of spoken vocabulary to describe emotions, and learn to express their own subtle emotions accurately and clearly using non-verbal communication. They also need to learn to read the subtle emotion cues in the non-verbal communication of others.

Affective education also includes working on the connection between thoughts, feelings, and behavior, and learning how to conceptualize emotions and change the perception of various situations. Another component of affective education is explaining why we have specific emotions, especially anxiety, as a natural survival mechanism, and describing the parts of the brain involved in emotional experiences.

Cognitive restructuring

The subsequent stage is *cognitive restructuring*, that is, learning how the brain can manage intense emotions, and includes a schedule of activities to practice new cognitive emotion expression and management skills in real-life situations.

THE EMOTIONAL TOOLBOX

From an early age, children understand that a toolbox contains a variety of different tools to repair a machine or fix a household problem. The psychologist, therapist, or parent works with the child to identify different types of "tools" to fix the problems associated with negative emotions, especially anxiety, sadness, and anger. The range of tools can be divided into those that:

- quickly and constructively release emotional energy
- slowly reduce emotional energy
- improve thinking and cognitive control of emotions.

PHYSICAL TOOLS

A hammer can represent tools or actions that physically release emotional energy. A picture of a hammer is drawn on a large sheet of paper and the child suggests safe and appropriate physical activities. For young children, this may include such activities as going for a run, bouncing on the trampoline, or going on a swing. For older children, sports practice and dancing may be used to "let off steam" or release emotional energy.

RELAXATION TOOLS

Relaxation tools help to calm the person and lower the heart rate. A paintbrush could be used to illustrate this category of tools, and activities could include drawing, reading, and listening to music. Children with Asperger's syndrome often find that solitude is their most relaxing activity. They may need to retreat to a quiet, secluded sanctuary as an effective emotional repair mechanism. However, at school, it is very difficult to achieve solitude and the program may need to include opportunities to be briefly and safely alone during the school day. Young children may relax by using gentle rocking actions and engaging in a repetitive action. This can include manipulating an object such as a stress ball that has the same soothing qualities as an adult manipulating worry beads. A relaxation tool that is proving to be increasingly effective, especially with adolescents, is meditation.

SOCIAL TOOLS

This group of tools uses other people as a means of managing feelings. The goal is to find and be with someone (or an animal or pet) that can help change the mood. The social activity will need to be enjoyable and without the stress that can sometimes be associated with social interaction, especially when interacting with more than one other person. Remember the saying, "two's company, three's a crowd," especially for those who have Asperger's syndrome. However, there are some people, children and adults, who seem to have a natural ability to absorb the anguish of someone who has Asperger's syndrome, and time with such people can be incorporated into the CBT program to help manage emotions.

THINKING TOOLS

The child can nominate another type of implement, such as a wrench, to represent a category of tools that can be used to change thinking, improve knowledge, or challenge inappropriate beliefs. The child is encouraged to use his or her intellectual strength to control feelings using a variety of techniques. Self-talk can be used, such as, "I can control my feelings" or "I can stay calm" when under stress. The words are reassuring and encourage self-confidence and self-esteem.

SPECIAL INTEREST TOOLS

Children with Asperger's syndrome can experience intense pleasure when engaged in their special interest. The degree of enjoyment may be far in excess of other potentially pleasurable experiences. The child can be encouraged to engage in his or her interest as a means of restoring the emotional equilibrium—a counterbalance of pleasure, sometimes perceived as an "off switch." The activity can sometimes appear to be mesmerizing and dominating all thought, but this can be effective at excluding negative thoughts such as anxiety and anger, thus an effective "thought blocker." When the child with Asperger's syndrome is very distressed, the most effective emotional restoratives are usually solitude and becoming totally absorbed in the special interest.

MEDICATION

Medication is sometimes prescribed for children with Asperger's syndrome to manage emotions. If the child is showing clear signs of a diagnosable anxiety disorder or a clinical depression (which may be expressed as episodes of intense anger, irritability, or apathy), then medication may be recommended. However, it is important to ensure that medication is not the only tool we add to the Emotional Toolbox.

CBT TO EXPRESS AFFECTION

Within families and friendships, there is an expectation that there will be a mutually enjoyable, reciprocal, and beneficial regular exchange of words and gestures that express affection. One of the early signs that clinicians use to diagnose an ASD in an infant or young child is a lack of appearing to be comforted by affection when distressed. As a typical child matures, there is an intuitive understanding of the type, duration, and degree of affection appropriate for both the situation and person. Even children of under two years know that words and gestures of affection are perhaps the most effective emotional repair mechanism for themselves and for someone who is sad.

Unfortunately, for some children with an ASD, a hug can be experienced as an uncomfortable and restricting physical sensation, and the child may soon learn not to cry, as crying will elicit a "squeeze" from someone. Children with an ASD such as Asperger's syndrome may also not recognize the social conventions regarding affection; for example, the child might express and expect in return the same degree of affection with a teacher as they would with their mother.

In general, a child with Asperger's syndrome may enjoy a very brief and low intensity expression of affection, but become confused or overwhelmed when greater levels of expression are experienced or expected. However, the reverse can occur for some children with Asperger's syndrome, where they need almost excessive amounts of affection, sometimes for reassurance but also for a sensory experience, and often express affection that is too intense or immature.

The child's rare use of gestures and words of affection can be lamented by parents and friends, who may feel affection-deprived and not demonstrably liked or loved. We now have CBT programs to help children who have Asperger's syndrome express and enjoy affection with family members and friends (see Further Reading section).

Learning abilities and styles

Profile of learning abilities

Children with Asperger's syndrome usually have an unusual and uneven profile of learning abilities, as well as an unusual learning style, which can be confusing for teachers. Some children with Asperger's syndrome can be quite talented in terms of reading, spelling, or mathematical and mechanical abilities, while others can have specific learning problems in these areas.

While the child's IQ may be within the normal or even superior range, some individual test scores in the profile of intellectual abilities may be within the intellectual disability range, or a specific component of the school curriculum may seem unexpectedly incomprehensible for the child—for example, he or she may be talented in mathematics, but have great difficulty with algebra. An assessment of intellectual ability on a standardized intelligence scale and an assessment of academic abilities can provide invaluable information for teachers and parents with regard to the child's learning style and lead to effective remedial programs for areas of conspicuous difficulties.

Learning style

Verbalizers and visualizers

Teaching is primarily a social and conversational activity, which is not the optimum or natural way of learning for those who have an ASD, due to their associated specific difficulties with social communication. If the child with Asperger's syndrome has a relatively higher verbal IQ, he or she may be described as a "verbalizer," and the child may succeed academically by reading about the subject rather than participating in the social/ conversational and group-based classroom activities.

If the child is a "visualizer," learning may be facilitated by silent demonstrations, films, and diagrams, and the advice that "a picture is worth a thousand words." Such children can be natural engineers. However, the child may have in his or her mind the "picture" or solution to a problem, but not the thousand words to provide an explanation. Such children can have difficulty converting thoughts into speech. For both groups, remedial programs may be more successful if the curriculum or concept is explained on a computer screen rather than in the social and linguistic context of the classroom.

Fear of making a mistake

Children and adolescents who have Asperger's syndrome often have a pathological fear of making a mistake or failure, and some activities may be refused if there is the possibility of not being perfect. Such children can be very sensitive about appearing stupid to the teacher, and especially to peers, and value intelligence highly in themselves and others. A mistake challenges their self-perception and value system. Social Stories™ can be used to explain the importance of learning more from errors than success, and that the child is not stupid for making a mistake.

Encouraging motivation

A useful motivational tool is to appeal to the child's intellectual vanity, replacing personal delight with unemotional comments that the work indicates how smart he or she is. The usual motivation of praise from the teacher may not be as effective as with typical children. This approach may help overcome a common problem: the motivation of the child with Asperger's syndrome for classroom activities that are not intrinsically interesting.

Adaptations to examinations and tests

The child may need extra time, supervision, and the facility to type rather than write answers and essays in an exam or test. Otherwise, they may lose marks on timed tests because of difficulties due to problems with working quickly, being pedantic and too thorough, being distracted by details, and by handwriting problems.

The teacher or parent may have to act as an "executive secretary" with guidance and allowances for problems with "executive skills" (see Chapter 3). Without this help, there may also be problems with executive functioning, especially organizational, planning, and time management skills that affect school projects and homework.

A one-track mind

The child with Asperger's syndrome may prefer to follow his or her own idiosyncratic ideas and solutions rather than copying the other children, or heeding the advice of the teacher. In class, they are notorious for being very rigid in thinking style—a "one-track mind." There can also be difficulties switching tracks when a strategy or solution is not successful (flexibility in thinking), and problems losing their train of thought when interrupted. Teachers will need to explain that there are many ways to solve some problems, and that the smart thing to do is to remain calm, try another way, observe the other children, or ask for help.

Special interests

Highly restricted, repetitive patterns of behavior, interests or activities are an essential part of the diagnostic criteria for ASD. These characteristics can develop in young children with an ASD as early as age two to three years, and may commence with a preoccupation with parts of objects. The interest can be spinning the wheels of toy cars or manipulating electrical switches. The next—or first stage for some children with Asperger's syndrome—is a fascination with and attachment to a specific category of objects and the accumulation of as many examples as possible. Sometimes the collections comprise items typically acquired by other children, such as unusual stones, but some can be quite eccentric, such as drain covers.

The child's play can also be somewhat eccentric in that he or she can pretend to be the special interest. One child had a special interest in toilets and in the playground pretended to be a blocked toilet. Another child, attending a special "costume day" at school (where children typically chose film characters or animals) went as a washing machine—his special interest.

The next stage is for children to acquire information regarding a topic or concept. Common topics or concepts are vehicles (especially trains), animals, and electronics. Some of the interests are developmentally appropriate and typical of their peers, such as Thomas the Tank Engine, dinosaurs, castles, and computer games, while other interests can be unusual, such as vacuum cleaners and alarm systems. The reason for the interest is usually idiosyncratic, and not necessarily because the topic is popular with peers, or is the "currency" between friends.

The duration of a specific interest can be from hours to decades, but the focus of the interest invariably changes, at a time dictated by the child, and is replaced by another special interest that is also the choice of the child, not a parent or teacher. The complexity and number of interests vary according to the child's developmental level and intellectual capacity. Over time, there is a progression to multiple and more abstract or complex interests, such as periods of history, the periodic table or specific countries/cultures.

The special interests of girls

Clinical experience suggests that boys and girls with Asperger's syndrome differ in the type of interest they choose. The girls can develop an intense interest in dolls, animals, and fiction. Again, some of the interests are age- and gender-appropriate but unusual in their intensity. The interest in dolls can lead to a huge collection of dolls but a preference to play with dolls alone rather than with a peer. The doll play can include detailed re-enactments of scenes from the child's daily life to retrospectively analyze social situations. The interest in animals can be to such an intensity that the child acts being the animal, and if the interest is horses, may want to sleep in a stable. The interest in fiction can include collecting, and reading many times, the novels of a favorite author, such as J.K. Rowling, and an interest in classical literature, such as Shakespeare's plays and the stories of Charles Dickens or Mark Twain. This stems not from a desire to achieve success at school in English literature, but from a genuine interest in the great authors and their works. The girl may also appreciate being able to actually read what a person may be thinking or feeling, especially when having difficulty "reading" body language and facial expressions in real life.

Adolescent interests

In the teenage years the interests can evolve to include electronics and computers, fantasy literature, science fiction, and sometimes a fascination with a particular person. All of these mirror the interests of peers, but, again, the intensity and focus is unusual. There can be a natural ability to understand computer languages, graphics, and advanced computer programming. The interest in fantasy literature and fantasy figures can be so intense that the people may develop their own role-play games and remarkably detailed drawing skills based on their special interest. There can also be a fascination with a particular character—mythical, historical, or real. When the interest is focused on a real person, it can be interpreted as a teenage "crush," although the intensity can lead to accusations of stalking and harassment.

Why does the child develop a special interest?

We are only just beginning to understand what may be the cause of the development of special interests. Parents of children with Asperger's syndrome, and autobiographies written by adults with an ASD, have described how an initial source of fear can develop into a special interest. An acute auditory sensitivity to the noise of a vacuum cleaner, for example, can lead to a fascination with the different types of vacuum cleaner and how they work; a fear of the sound of thunder may become an interest in weather systems and knowing when they are likely to occur. The child's intelligent and practical way of reducing the fear is to learn about the cause of his or her anxiety.

It is also fascinating that some interests are triggered by situations associated with a pleasurable experience. The interest is commemorative, linked to a memory of a pleasurable time or event, such as a visit to a theme park or science museum. Thinking about the interest can act as the "antidote" to negative thoughts or experiences. When we conduct an assessment of the pleasures in the child's life, children with Asperger's syndrome often value time engaged in their special interest more than almost any other pleasure, including interpersonal experiences.

Another characteristic is that the child is almost mesmerized by the activity. This can be used as a means of preventing the intrusion of negative thoughts—a form of thought blocking when feeling anxious or depressed.

Reducing and using the special interest

While the motivation for the child with Asperger's syndrome is to increase his or her access to the interest, perhaps at the expense of other activities, the motivation for parents and teachers is to reduce the duration of the access to enable the child to engage in a wider range of activities. This is particularly important when the interest appears to virtually exclude social interaction with family members at home and peers at school, or affects the completion of homework assignments. What are the strategies that can reduce the time spent engaged in the interest? Can special interests serve a constructive purpose?

Controlled access

The problem may not be the activity itself but the duration and dominance over other interests. Some success can be achieved by limiting the time available using a clock or timer. When the allotted time is over, the activity must cease and the child can be actively encouraged to pursue other interests. Reassurance can be given that there will be another scheduled time for the chosen interest. The temptation to continue the activity will be quite strong, so the new activity may have to be in another room or outside. The replacement activity also needs to be something the child enjoys, even if it is not as enjoyable as the special interest. The approach is to ration access, and to actively encourage a wider range of interests.

Part of the controlled access program can be to allocate specific social or "quality" time to pursue the interest as a social activity. A parent or teacher has a schedule of regular times to talk about or jointly explore the interest. The adult ensures that they are not going to be distracted, and both parties view the experience as enjoyable. I have found that such sessions can be an opportunity to improve my own knowledge of such interesting topics as the *Guinness Book of Records*, the Titanic, and *Star Wars* and Dr. Who. I am then able to talk with some authority and achieve respect from the children I meet with Asperger's syndrome who have the same interests.

Encouraging motivation

Children with Asperger's syndrome have significant motivation and prolonged attention span when involved with their special interest. The treatment strategy is to incorporate the special interest in the classroom activity or to use access to the interest as a reward. For example, if the young child has an interest in Thomas the Tank Engine, there is a wide range of merchandise that incorporates the engines in reading books for different reading ages, mathematical activities, and writing and drawing. If the young child is interested in geography and flags in particular, he or she could count flags rather than the conventional items being counted by peers.

The interest can simply be used as a reward. Completion of allocated tasks in class results in free time to pursue the interest. For example, if he completes the ten addition problems within ten minutes, he has earned ten minutes on his computer. Access to the interest is a remarkably potent reward. This strategy does require the teacher to be more flexible in the presentation of the class tasks, the curriculum, and reward systems. However, the benefits can be quite extraordinary to the child who can widen his or her knowledge base, demonstrate intellectual ability, and attain prizes and certificates of achievement through constructive utilization of the special interest.

Some parents have used the removal of access to the interest as a punishment for tasks not completed or misbehavior. While this strategy can sometimes be an effective component of a home-based behavior management program, there is a risk that temporary removal could become a trigger for extreme frustration and subsequent aggressive or agitated behavior. This strategy may be counterproductive in a behavior or emotion management program. This is because the interest has many functions, including being a pleasurable experience and energy restorative, creating a feeling of genuine achievement, and managing emotions by being a thought blocker. The special interest is perceived as an essential component of life by the person who has Asperger's syndrome.

A means of making friends

"What makes a good friend?" For many typical children the reply is, "We like the same things." Shared interests can be a source of friendship. I know a child with Asperger's syndrome who has a remarkable interest in and knowledge of ants. His class peers tolerated his enthusiasm and monologues on ants, but he was not regarded as a popular choice of companion. He was learning a range of friendship skills, such as waiting, sharing, compliments, and empathy. When he expressed these skills, they were achieved by intellectual effort and support and were perceived by others as somewhat contrived and artificial. He had few genuine friends. By chance, another child with Asperger's syndrome lived close by. He also had an interest in ants. There was an arranged meeting and the result amazed their parents and teachers. They were companions on ant-finding expeditions, made a joint ant study, and regularly contacted each other with their latest ant-related discoveries. However, when observing their interactions, there was a natural fluency and quality to their social skills. They waited patiently, listened attentively, showed empathy, and gave compliments at a level not observed with their peers. Parents may consider, therefore, some social engineering using the child's special interest to encourage prospective friendships. Local parent support groups can include the names and addresses of group members, but also the special interests of their son or daughter for the possibility of an arranged but potentially successful friendship.

Can the signs of Asperger's syndrome become less conspicuous over time?

Yes, they can. Recent longitudinal studies and my own clinical experience have confirmed that around 10–15 percent of children who have a diagnosis of Asperger's syndrome in early childhood can progress in their early adult years to such a mild and inconspicuous level of expression of ASD that, to use the terminology in DSM-5, the person no longer fulfills criterion D, namely, "Symptoms cause a clinically significant impairment in social, occupational or other important areas of current functioning" (APA 2013, p.50).

The child with Asperger's syndrome has a brain that is wired differently, not necessarily defectively. They do not have the depth of intuitive ability in social communication and social interaction as their peers, and engage in restricted, repetitive patterns of behavior. However, over time—and with understanding and guidance—the adolescent and young adult who had clear signs of Asperger's syndrome in early childhood can gradually learn how to relate to others and to manage and limit restricted and repetitive behavior. Some children with Asperger's syndrome can eventually learn what to do and say, such that they are able to achieve both a successful career and long-term personal relationships. It is possible to solve the social puzzle, using intellect and guidance, and reach a point where the signs of Asperger's syndrome are no longer clinically significant. The prognosis for those who have Asperger's syndrome is now much better than we once thought.

CHAPTER 7

Anxiety and Obsessive-Compulsive Disorders

"Susan worries so much! All of us used to worry about a test the next day, but she worries about it for days in advance. In fact, she seems to worry about lots of things. She's even worried about next year. She tells me that it doesn't make sense, but she just can't help thinking about this stuff. I used to think that she avoided school because she just didn't like it. Now, I'm beginning to think that it's just too painful for her. In order to leave the house now for school, she goes through this little ritual of touching the door three times. It's just so sad to watch."

Generalized anxiety disorder (GAD)

Anxiety disorders share the common thread of excessive fear and anxiety that exceed the person's ability to comfortably control them, often leading to avoidance behaviors. According to the American Psychiatric Association's DSM-5 definition of generalized anxiety disorder (APA 2013), the fear and anxieties must be sufficiently severe to interfere with functioning in life. The worries are about multiple things, occur most days, and feel difficult to control. In addition, there are physical symptoms such as insomnia, tiredness, restlessness, irritableness, tense muscles, or concentrating difficulties.

Prevalence rates for GAD range are 2–9% for girls, and 1–4% for boys (Bernstein and Layne 2004). Overall, there seems to be overlapping roles of genetic temperament, parenting style, support systems, and life events in the development of GAD.

Children with GAD also have a two-thirds risk of having at least one of the other conditions of the syndrome mix described in this book, and these problems typically exacerbate each other. In particular, children with GAD have a one in four chance of having attention deficit hyperactivity disorder (ADHD) (Bernstein and Layne 2004).

According to the current theory of GAD, there is an imbalance in the loop between the brain's cortex and primitive centers for sensory input and emotion. Sometimes, these emotion centers get triggered without the conscious part of the brain even being "notified" of why, leading to the (unfair) situation where we may experience nervousness, but not be consciously aware of what set it off.

Obviously, all of us worry to some degree. In fact, it would be hard to survive without some measure of worry. For example, why would we store extra food today if we weren't worried about being hungry during the winter? Why would we build a house now if we weren't worried about getting cold or wet? Why would we study if there were no test tomorrow? Indeed, there is an evolutionary advantage to appropriate amounts of worry.

So what is too much worry? We can distinguish generalized anxiety disorder (GAD) from normal childhood worries as follows:

- GAD kids worry about lots of things (six or more) at a time; typical kids only worry about one thing at time.

- GAD kids with sufficient insight find the worry useless, unwelcome, and "alien"; typical kids may realize that small amounts of worry help them perform better.

- GAD kids usually *recognize* that they tend to worry more about things than their peers.

- GAD kids *anticipate* future events and worry about (or try to avoid) them well in advance; typical kids worry about *immediate* problems.

- GAD worries are stronger, more painful, and more disruptive. GAD kids worry about things that other children find trivial.

- GAD kids may have insomnia, poor concentration, irritability, or appear on edge.

- GAD kids often have bodily complaints such as headaches, abdominal pain, etc.

Sometimes, GAD kids can present as perfectionists. Although "perfectionism" is not recognized per se as a neuropsychiatric disorder, it certainly needs to be considered here as a type of anxiety. The school psychologist Dr. Kenneth Shore distinguishes between healthy striving for excellence and perfectionism as follows (Shore 2002):

- Striving for excellence:
  ◦ Reaches for challenges.
  ◦ Derives pleasure from the process.
  ◦ Attributes success to hard work.
  ◦ A failure means weakness in one area.
  ◦ Celebrates accomplishments.
- Perfectionism:
  ◦ Avoids challenges.
  ◦ Focuses mostly on the end product.
  ◦ Attributes success to luck.
  ◦ Failure means weakness as a person.
  ◦ Celebrates avoidance of failure.

In many nations, there has been a strong trend towards an increasingly educationally based and technologically driven culture. Contemporary society often places an extremely high premium on the value of education, more so than ever before. Now, many parents are preoccupied not just by trying to have their children attend college, but it must be a "good" college. Parents worry about whether their children will be able to support themselves. Unfortunately, this has all created a generation of young people who feel overwhelmed and pushed much of the time. These overscheduled and overly competitive children often do not get enough "down time," the value of which is often overlooked. Children need to learn to regulate themselves, and appreciate their own needs. A balanced lifestyle is harder to learn than might be imagined.

Childhood anxiety is easy to miss

A striking feature of childhood anxiety is that often no one else knows about the problem. In fact, even the mothers of anxious children do not recognize the problem about half of the time (Bernstein and Layne 2004)—a surprising statistic since mothers often know more about their child than the child does herself.

Interestingly, many children with anxiety disorders intuitively appreciate that they tend to, "worry more about things than other children their age." Often, directly asking a child if she worries more than other kids will allow her to feel comfortable talking about it. The usual triggers are poor school performance (they feel less smart than classmates), a loss (death, illness), parental discord, witnessing violence directed towards themselves or others, or concerns over personal appearance (obesity, acne, height).

Sleep disturbances are an important physiologic window into anxiety disorders. Insomnia (commonly defined as difficulty regularly falling asleep within 20 minutes after your head is on the pillow) is a very frequent symptom. Early morning awakening, such as at 3am, and difficulty falling asleep again, are also common manifestations of anxiety. This may all lead to subsequent daytime sleepiness, which can contribute to poor school performance. (Note that loud snoring with obstructive sleep apnea can also cause daytime sleepiness and attention problems, but is not usually associated with insomnia.)

Since it is so easy to fail to recognize the anxiety disorder, we must always think about it when faced with a child who seems to only present with bodily complaints, avoidance, inattention, or irritability—and we frequently need to directly ask the child about it. Questions to be answered include the following:

- Does the child worry or ask the parents for reassurance almost all days?

- Are age-appropriate activities avoided or only done with a parent?

- Are there bodily complaints such as stomachaches?

- Are there daily, repetitive rituals?

(Tannock 2009, p.146)

Other anxiety disorders

When diagnosing anxiety disorders, we must look to see if a more specific anxiety disorder fits the child better than generalized anxiety disorder. Other DSM-5 anxiety disorders are briefly described below.

- *Separation anxiety* involves anxiety about being or becoming separated from home or "attachment figures" (such as parents), including fear that something might happen to either party causing the child to be alone. Separation anxiety is often an early marker for other future anxiety disorders.

- *Selective mutism* is when a child is perfectly capable of speaking when in a comfortable setting, but consistently fails to talk in certain other social settings such as school.

- *Specific phobia* is when the fear and avoidance symptoms are limited to one or more specific situations or things, such as animals, heights, or airplanes.

- *Social anxiety disorder (social phobia)* is when the anxiety/fear is centered around social situations where the child feels subject to scrutiny/evaluation by others. The child fears she will be negatively evaluated. In children, this anxiety must extend to relations with peers, not just with adults. This impairing reaction leads to avoidance or the experience of intense fear or anxiety. Only a small fraction of people who identify themselves as "shy" actually meet criteria for social anxiety disorder.

- *Panic disorder* is marked by repeated, *unexpected* panic attacks accompanied by significant worry about their recurrence and fears of losing control or being ill; or accompanied by maladaptive avoidance behaviors. There may additionally be *expected* (predictable) panic attacks. Panic disorder must be distinguished from the term "panic attack." Panic attacks—expected or unexpected—can occur as part of many psychiatric disorders, such as any of the anxiety disorders, depression, bipolar, etc. The presence of panic attacks usually belies a more severe degree of such underlying psychiatric disorders. Their presence can be noted diagnostically as a "specifier" tag added to the primary diagnosis; for example, "separation anxiety with panic attacks."

- *"Agorophobia"* denotes fear/anxiety in at least two of the following environments: being in enclosed space; being in open spaces; being in crowds; being alone outside of the house; or using public transit (e.g., buses or trains). There is accompanying fear of inability to escape from such places should panic set in.

- *Unspecified anxiety disorder* refers to anxiety that causes functional impairment but does not fully meet criteria for any of the anxiety conditions above.

Obsessive-compulsive disorder (OCD)

Anxiety or apprehension is also at the root of the obsessive-compulsive disorder (OCD) loop. The person has a thought → anxiety that the loop is happening again → more thoughts. For example, an accountant might start to wonder if he made a mistake on a client's taxes. He knows that he did not actually make a significant mistake, but becomes afraid that these worries will keep coming back. The fear of ruining his whole weekend over these stupid worries makes him even more anxious, and the loop recurs, until he finally goes back to the office to check. (Unfortunately, the pleasant yet short-lived relief from the fear, that results from such checking again, reinforces the likelihood that the whole cycle will start again.) There is a fear of fear powering the cycle. Without the anxiety, there is nothing driving the loop. In fact, an obsession is basically an irrational, recurrent anxiety. OCD and anxiety are basically part of a single anxiety/OCD spectrum.

Obsessions are repetitive *thoughts or urges* that are experienced by the person as unwelcome and basically senseless. The person feels compelled to try to ignore or neutralize the anxiety caused by these useless thoughts. *Compulsions* are the *behaviors or mental acts* that the person feels obliged to carry out in order to ward off the anxiety caused by the obsessions. These behaviors—such as counting, touching, rechecking, or repeating words silently—may need to be carried out according to rigid rules. The behaviors are clearly excessive and unrealistic in their ability to head off the dreaded worry. For example, in order to ensure a safe bus ride, a child may feel the need to say "goodbye" exactly four times before she leaves the house. Logically speaking, though, this act won't really affect the safety record of the bus. This is one of the distinguishing factors between OCD and other anxiety disorders. In generalized anxiety disorder, the worries relate to real-life concerns, such as finances or making friends, whereas in OCD, the behaviors are magical, odd, or just don't make sense. The presence of compulsive acts is another feature of OCD that distinguishes it from other anxiety disorders.

The adult—at some point—recognizes that this is all unreasonable or excessive. Children may not reach this realization, and usually do not explicitly spell out obsessions or compulsions unless specifically asked about them. Note that these problems must be severe enough to interfere with the quality of life before a diagnosis can be made, and may extort more than one hour per day from their "host."

Typical OCD domains of concern include:

- cleaning (including fear of contamination)

- counting or symmetry (e.g., need to touch on the left if touched on the right)

- harm (to self or others, perhaps with the need for repeated checking to prevent that harm)

- taboo thoughts (including religious, aggressive, or sexual unwanted thoughts).

When OCD is being considered, attention should also be paid to the possible presence of tics, which run up to a 30% lifetime risk (APA 2013, p.238), any other element of the "syndrome mix" in this text, and particular OCD-related disorders such as:

- *trichotillomania* (hair-pulling)

- *skin picking disorder*, or

- *body dysmorphic disorder* (perception of defects in physical appearance).

Treatment

Inside the classroom (and at home as well)
Let the child know that you understand

If you are having trouble watching these obsessive-compulsive rituals, imagine how uncomfortable it must be to struggle with them directly. *Anxiety/OCD can be very painful!* Let the child know that you understand how difficult these issues can be. Just knowing that the adult understands can be of great help.

Let her know that you recognize that by the time she gets to school, she may have already struggled with the stress of getting through her thoughts/rituals while trying to get to class on time. She may have stayed up late trying to perfect her work. There may have been fights between the child and her parents/siblings when she would not—or could not—comply with the others' needs. There may have been wrenching struggles over finding the "right" clothes, or with repetitive trips to the washroom.

Provide a safe, supportive environment

Shore (2002) suggests the following strategies for perfectionist children—which can be extrapolated to the anxiety disorders.

- The class should be conducive to taking academic risks.

- All attempts at achievement should be celebrated—not just the successful ones.

- Make the classroom a safe haven where mistakes are expected.

- Make sure goals are realistic and explicit.

- De-emphasize grades.

- Use humor.

- Encourage students to trust their own judgment, which is a more useful skill in the long run than the short-term success that comes from double-checking everything daily with the teacher.

- Teach: "We all make mistakes—that's why they put erasers on pencils."

Talk with students about their needs. Ask students for their ideas as to how you can assist them. Dr. Leslie Packer (2005) suggests the following strategies:

- Find out what things set off their worries/rituals, and work out ways to deal with those stimuli. For example, if trying to perfect handwriting is bothersome, then work out a practical solution—such as using a laptop, oral exams, providing breaks, or agreeing upon the amount of time for their written work.

- Recognize that *anxieties or OCD may silently interfere with work*. Sometimes, the anxieties or obsessions may cause silent, internal distractions. Keep an eye out for these hidden distractions as causes of the apparent symptoms of inattention, slow performance, or work avoidance. Alternatively, anxiety may cause excessive trips to the bathroom or school nurse.

- Ask the child whether she would like to be subtly refocused when she appears internally distracted by her worries.

- Allow *extra time* as needed. Extra time may be necessary when:

  ◦ internal distractions slow the work

  ◦ it will alleviate anxiety associated with finishing "on time"

  ◦ it will accommodate for rituals, such as having to write perfectly, repeatedly erase, or exactly fill in the circles.

Agree upon *limits for perfectionism* by using the following strategies:

- Make a contract with the child to hand in work after an agreed upon limit of work time, or after a certain amount of rechecking.

- Avoid reinforcing the perfectionism that comes from praising it. Rather, reinforce reasonable effort and its resultant imperfections.

- Work out an *"escape route."* Pre-arrange that the child may leave the room when she feels the need. Perhaps a trip to the bathroom will resettle the nerves. Or, perhaps, a trip when needed to the school guidance counselor or psychologist might be agreed upon in advance.

- *Educate peers* who are teasing the child. Children with anxiety disorders often try to hide their problems from their peers—a stressful process, at best. Even so, the rituals may be so uncontrollable that even friends cannot tolerate them. Have a session about accepting diversity, and educate fellow students about anxiety/OCD. This would probably need to be done in consultation with the child, family, and mental health professionals. The Obsessive Compulsive Foundation has materials of great use to families, teachers, and patients at www.ocfoundation.org.

Professional treatment outside the classroom
Cognitive behavioral therapy (CBT)

Cognitive behavioral therapy (CBT) utilizes a combination of cognitive (thinking strategies) and behavioral strategies (such as pushing through the fears) to give the child and her family a "toolbox" of techniques that empower the child to overcome her ritual/fear. A particularly powerful type of CBT is called Exposure and Response Prevention (ERP). In ERP, the patient is exposed to doses of the feared situation and is restricted from carrying out the typical compulsive response. The patient thereby discovers that the feared activity has no real power over her—it was a false alarm—and can be tolerated without resorting to the compulsion previously used to obtain transient relief from the fear. A counselor, such as a psychologist, usually provides this type of training. CBT skills might include the following elements:

- Teaching well-intentioned family members to avoid reinforcing anxieties/OCD rituals when they constantly make accommodations for the child's areas of difficulty.

- Guiding the child to resist the urge to perform a ritual—and thereby letting the child know that he can tolerate and break through the fear that he thought resisting the urge would provoke (ERP). This helps diminish the fear of fear that fueled the OCD cycle.

- Avoiding "awfulizing" the process where one always exaggerates the importance of an event and expects an unreasonably horrible outcome. For example, a child may think that if he is late for school, he'll get an "F" and will no longer be able to go to college. He needs reminders that if he is late, then he'll get...a late slip. Not the end of the world.

- Learning how to reframe one's attitude. For example, learning to see events as challenging opportunities rather than threats.

- Learning the process of thought blocking, where an intrusive thought is deliberately replaced by a pleasant one. For example, whenever the child is about to worry about a test, he is taught to instead imagine that he is relaxing at the beach.

Such cognitive behavioral therapies can be very effective for anxiety/OCD spectrum disorders—even more effective than medication. CBT also teaches skills that may last a lifetime (although booster sessions are often helpful). For these reasons CBT is often felt to be the preferred first line of treatment, if there is a therapist trained in CBT with children in your area.

Medication

If CBT is not available locally, is proving ineffective, or if the child cannot even try CBT due to severe anxiety/OCD, then medication may be required. The mainstays of the medication treatment of anxiety/OCD disorders are the selective serotonin reuptake inhibitors (SSRIs) such as Prozac (fluoxetine). They are remarkably helpful for this indication, and may make the strategies above more likely to be successful. Some authorities, though, worry that taking away the "pain" of the anxiety with medication may circumvent the child's desire to use the cognitive approaches above. Note that although stimulants have been felt to be contraindicated in ADHD with co-morbid anxiety disorder, recent evidence actually shows that one out of five such children have meaningful reduction in their anxiety when stimulants are used for their ADHD (Tannock 2009, p.143). See Chapter 14 for more information about medications.

CHAPTER 8

Sensory Integration Dysfunction (SID or SPD)

Martin L. Kutscher, MD with Joelle Glick

"Jane, come over and look at this! It's a great view from the top of the Empire State Building! If you come close enough to the edge, you can almost look straight down! Don't worry. The window will keep you from falling. You're perfectly safe."

Some of us seek such sensory input. Others will flee from it at any cost. All minds have equal rights, but all minds do not have the same response to stimuli.

How the brain works (in four paragraphs)

The brain is a problem-solving machine. The problems come in the form of sensory input. Our brain collects that information from our sensory receptors, integrates it all, evaluates its importance, forms a plan, and executes our solution. Problem solved. It is time for the next one.

We are most familiar with our external sensory input—*sight, taste, hearing, touch,* and *smell.* There are also internal senses that regulate our bodies without our even being aware of it. These internal senses include *tactile sense,* which includes all the information that we process through our skin (such as being able to identify something we hold in our hand—like a key—just by feeling it); *vestibular sense*, which monitors our position in space through gravity and motion; and *proprioceptive sense*, which informs us of our body position and body parts through the muscles, ligaments, and joints even without looking.

When stimulated, sensory receptors send an electrical current to the brain via a nerve. We only "know" what type of stimulus happened because the neurons from different sensory receptors go to different parts of the brain.

In addition to these objective reality reports that are sent to our brain, the brain's primitive limbic system also applies an emotional tag to each event. For example, some of us find that scrambled eggs evoke the memory of a nutritious, warm family breakfast. Some children find that scrambled eggs evoke from the limbic system the feeling of snake saliva. Everyone does not experience life in the same manner. We each have different ways of garnering information and reacting to it. Most of such sensory processing is subconscious. Only a selective portion is explicitly under our deliberate control. Once the stimulus is sensed and processed, the brain prepares and executes some sort of physical or other response.

What is sensory integration dysfunction (SID or SPD)?

Definitions

To begin with, *sensory integration* (SI) is defined as the process by which our brain interprets this information that we gather from our senses, and then outputs a meaningful response. For example, when someone gently pats you on the shoulder, your brain interprets the pleasant sensation of the hand on your back, and you calmly turn around to see who it is. *Sensory integration dysfunction (also referred to as sensory processing dysfunction—SPD)* is the brain's inability to process senses correctly or adaptively.

Dysfunction occurs when one or more of the links in the sensory network are in disequilibrium.

- Intake by the sensory system. The brain takes in too much (called *hypersensitivity*) or too little (called *hyposensitivity*) sensory information. Hypersensitive individuals will avoid stimuli that excessively arouse them. Hyposensitive individuals will either ignore the stimuli, or will crave stimuli in order to arouse themselves. In either case, information is not received at the correct volume level.

- Organization by the nervous system. Sensory data is either not received, received inconsistently, or disconnected from the correct sensory messages.

- Output of movement, speech, or emotion. Output problems can reflect a muscle control problem; or may be the result of faulty input or processing (i.e., garbage in; garbage out).

The following descriptions come largely from the landmark work, *The Out-of-Sync Child* by Sally Kranowitz (2005, 1998), which has made the whole area of SID accessible to modern readers. See also "Sensory integration dysfunction" in the Further Reading section.

Hypersensitivity (or "over-responsive," i.e., "oh, no!")

The brain of a hypersensitive child registers sensations too intensely—inducing an "Oh, no!" response. For example, most of us find a friend's voice to be soothing. Imagine, though, if that voice came in AT TOO LOUD A VOLUME, AND THERE SEEMED TO BE CONSTANT YELLING. Similarly, a child might be overwhelmed and run away from a light touch or a kiss on the cheek. He might defend himself from others, placing a physical barrier between himself and his surroundings in order to avoid stimuli. It is not unusual for hypersensitive children to respond to a minor scrape as if it were a life-threatening wound. They may even react to someone else's hurt feelings as if they were their own horrible experience. The hypersensitive child is often distractible because he is always paying attention to stimuli, regardless of importance.

Sometimes, the threatening nature of these stimuli to the child is easy to recognize. Other times, the child may not voice the problem, and it is subtler. All we may notice is that the child avoids certain situations, or may even seem inexplicably uncooperative, aggravated, or irritated.

Hyposensitivity (or "under-responsive," i.e., "ho, hum" or craves "more!")

The brain of a hyposensitive child interprets sensations less intensely than normal. This can lead to either ignoring the sensation (such as a "ho, hum" attitude towards a messy face), or the child may be very "touchy feely" in order to satisfy his craving for "more!" sensations. He may crash into objects or people because either he craves the sensation, he lacks proper motor control, he does not perceive the sensation until it is too late to move out of the way, or the crash doesn't bother him. The hyposensitive child enjoys wallowing in the mud or hanging upside down. He might fall off a bike and then get right back on without crying. Many hyposensitive children will appear tired or sleepy. They might have trouble interpreting normal social, non-verbal cues. For instance, the child may not comprehend a parent or teacher's scream. He might misinterpret another person's frown, and not react appropriately.

What about both?

Some children exhibit both hypersensitive and hyposensitive characteristics. The brain of a child who displays both characteristics cannot correctly modulate senses. His over- and under-sensitivity to stimuli may depend on the time of the day or the nature and intensity of the stimulus. This child is often difficult to get under control because it is unclear how and when to help him.

Categories of SID

Sensory integration dysfunctions have been classified into three categories.

Sensory modulation problems

The above over-responsive, under-responsive, and craving conditions have been dubbed "sensory modulation" disorders, since they share a common thread of poor regulation of sensory stimuli.

These problems are the main focus of this chapter.

Sensory discrimination problems

"Sensory discrimination problems" denotes trouble distinguishing one sensation from another (such as trouble telling where one is being touched), or correctly determining the significance of a sensation (such as correctly interpreting the significance of an injury).

Sensory-based motor problems

"Sensory-based motor problems" denotes either a "Postural Disorder" (such as difficulty maintaining proper muscle tone, maintaining proper posture, coordinating bilateral muscle movements, or settling on a hand preference), or "Dyspraxia" (such as difficulty with putting together a sequence of movements like brushing your teeth, with fine motor control of the mouth when eating or talking, or with fine motor control of the hands when writing).

Common symptoms

Each child will have different symptoms depending on the type of SID. For example, one child may be hypersensitive to touch and movement, while another child may be hyposensitive to touch and hypersensitive to movement. The following list includes common symptoms that occur under each category of SID.

A child who is:

- *hypersensitive to touch, taste, or textures* might: complain about discomfort caused by shirt tags, sock seams, turtlenecks, tight clothing, and rough-textured clothing; be a picky eater, prefer crunchy or soft foods, and dislike lumpy or sticky foods (tomato sauce or rice); refuse to have hair shampooed, combed, or brushed; withdraw from being touched; use fingertips (rather than the whole hand) to hold and investigate objects; avoid messy play with mud, sand, finger-paints, and glue

- *hyposensitive to touch, taste, or textures* may: crave deep hugs; be unresponsive to cuts, shots, bruises, or scrapes; seem unaware of touch unless it is intense; be unaware of a runny nose, or a dirty mouth; fail to realize he has dropped something; appear aggressive around other children because he does not comprehend the pain that the other children are feeling. Alternatively, the hyposensitive child may respond by craving spicy or crunchy foods in order to get adequate stimulation

- *hypersensitive to movement* may: dislike playground activities such as swinging, sliding, spinning, jumping, or climbing ramps, or jungle-gym equipment; feel uncomfortable while riding on an escalator or in an elevator; experience car or motion sickness; avoid taking risks, and appear slow moving or hesitant; have trouble learning how to climb or descend stairs or hills

- *hyposensitive to movement* might: enjoy (crave "more") continuous and forceful swinging, hanging upside down, and spinning; appear fidgety in class, unable to stay in his seat; enjoy the scarier rides at amusement parks; fail to become dizzy after strong spinning; or enjoy seesaws and trampolines more than other children.

A child who has:

- *low muscle tone* may: have a floppy body; lay her head on the table, lie on the floor, or slouch in a chair; have difficulty opening doors; tire easily (note: low muscle tone, in this case, does not indicate a problem with the child's muscles; the child's brain, however, is not sending the correct information to the muscles to provide the proper support and tension for daily activities)

- *poor fine motor control* might: curl his hands in loose fists or put his hands in his pockets; have difficulty manipulating scissors, markers, and utensils; have trouble buttoning shirts; use gestures to communicate if he has poor fine motor control of his tongue and lips.

SID, ADHD, autistic spectrum, anxiety, and learning disabilities

SID, attention deficit hyperactivity disorder (ADHD), autistic spectrum disorders (ASDs), and learning disabilities are separate but often co-existing disorders of the syndrome mix, which frequently elicit similar symptoms. A child might exhibit characteristics of ADHD or learning disabilities, but actually be suffering from SID, and vice versa. Many children with ASD have a significant degree of SID. In fact, increased or decreased sensitivity to sensory stimuli is actually one of the possible DSM-5 criteria for autism spectrum disorder. Despite many "look-alike" symptoms, the hallmarks of SID include a child's uncharacteristic behavior in response to touching, being touched, moving, and being moved.

Getting professional help

When and where

All of us have our likes and dislikes. That is totally normal. (As an example: "I don't like eggs.")

Sometimes, these likes and dislikes take on an unusual flair, but do not significantly interfere with function. We might call those "quirks." (For example: "I *never* eat eggs.")

At some point though, a person's likes and dislikes might cross the line and cause significant functional problems. (In this case: "I can't eat anywhere in the cafeteria because some of the other kids are eating eggs there.")

It is the latter group of problems—where likes and dislikes cause significant dysfunction—that the possibility of "sensory integration dysfunction" needs to be addressed professionally. The problems may be making the child miserable, or causing the life of people around him to be miserable. A screening checklist for parents and teachers can be found in Kranowitz (2005, pp.41–47).

In order to take advantage of the "plasticity" of a child's brain, significant sensory issues should ideally be identified early. Neural plasticity refers to the brain's capacity to change via the formation of new neuronal connections. The earlier the child gets help, the more likely he is to benefit from the treatment.

Observing good and bad behaviors at school and at home will help establish a pattern of the problem. Becoming aware of these patterns will be invaluable to yourself and the child. Make a chart of the incident, the time of day, and the child's complaint. This information will be extremely helpful in diagnosing the child and in determining a method for treatment.

Typical children build upon skills that they have learned and progress steadily into adulthood. Children with SID, however, may need the guided support of an occupational therapist (OT) to help them acquire the basic foundation for proper sensory integration. The therapy seems to facilitate the development of the child's nervous system, although well-documented research in the area is scarce.

You can find an OT through your school system, your doctor, your nearest children's or local hospital, or a professional organization such as The American Occupational Therapy Association (AOTA) at www.aota.org or the comprehensive SI site of the SPD Foundation at www.spdfoundation.net. Not all OTs are trained in SID.

Screening and evaluation
What is a screening?
A screening is often a short, informal approach taken to check whether or not a child has acquired certain skills. A screening will

often take place in a group setting, such as in a preschool. If any developmental problems have been suggested, the child's parents will be informed, and may be advised to get a full evaluation.

What is a full evaluation?

A full evaluation entails a thorough, individualized session typically performed by OTs trained in the area. They evaluate the child with the help of standardized tests, strict observation of the child, and a questionnaire filled out by the parents that will help establish patterns since birth. The professional will establish the child's strengths and weaknesses; where, when, and how often they occur; and the intensity and duration of their occurrence.

The therapist will make a diagnosis, write a report, and confer with the parents. Sometimes, the conclusion might be that time is the only remedy needed. Suggestions for games and activities at home might also be discussed. Other times, the professional will suggest individualized therapy sessions for the child. Since each child is different, the activities that the therapist suggests will vary from child to child.

Controversies regarding diagnosis and treatment

SID has not been as well recognized by the medical community as the other disorders in this book. There is still no medical classification of this disorder in the DSM-IV or DSM-5. Further a policy statement of the American Academy of Pediatrics (AAP 2012, pp.1186–1189) states:

> Because there is no universally accepted framework for diagnosis, sensory processing disorder generally should not be diagnosed... Difficulty tolerating or processing sensory information is a characteristic that may be seen in many developmental behavioral disorders, including ASDs, ADHD, developmental coordination disorders, and childhood anxiety disorders... Studies to date have not demonstrated that sensory integration dysfunction exists as a separate disorder distinct from these other developmental disabilities.

The AAP policy statement goes on to recommend that pediatricians discuss the limited evidence that occupational therapy is actually helpful; and if used there should be a clear methodology of testing the progress towards clearly defined goals—methodologies such as the use of rating scales or behavioral diaries. Families should be reminded that occupational therapy is a limited resource in most schools and insurance plans, and time limits should be set to discuss progress.

That all does not mean that the governing medical associations disagree that there are people who have sensory processing problems—just that these problems may be better understood as symptoms accompanying other disorders. Clearly, there *are* children who have sensory differences. We've all seen them. A recent validating study demonstrated that the electrodermal skin testing of 70 children with the diagnosis of SID showed a significantly greater response to auditory, visual, and movement stimuli when compared to ADHDers or neurotypical controls (Miller 2012).

Further impediments to therapy

Since it is difficult to do well-controlled, unbiased ("blind") research on the effectiveness of the varying treatments, it may be difficult to get school systems or health plans to cover unproven treatments. Also, many children resist the therapy— which is often a type of gradual desensitization. After all, we are asking them to slowly expose themselves more and more to the noxious stimuli—a therapy that they did not ask for, that may be particularly unpleasant, and whose long-term benefits may not be at all apparent to the child as he goes through the treatments. Therapy can be more enticing if it calls for activities that meet unfulfilled desires, such as the need for experiencing deep pressure or brushing.

Other types of therapy

Although most children with SID seem to benefit from occupational therapy, other more specific therapies might also be needed to help the problem. Some of these therapies include speech and language therapy, psychotherapy (if the child has become depressed and has a poor self-image), and physical therapy. Typically, physical therapy is used for gross motor problems or difficulties that involve the legs.

Treatment activities for home and school

Caregivers should provide the child with a balanced "sensory diet"—an OT should individually develop and supervise an appropriate program. The child's safety should always be paramount. When initiating a program with an occupational therapist, remember the following points:

☐ **Structure the activities**—have certain times during the day (such as before or after mealtimes) when the activities will take place.

☐ **Listen to the child**—let the child tell you which activities he wants. Allow him to tell you "more" or "less," but supervise carefully so that the child does not become overly aroused. Listen and watch for non-verbal clues during the activity to see which activities work the best.

☐ **Anticipate**—anticipating how the child will react, and what the child wants, will enable you to better respond to his needs.

☐ **Change the routine and environment**—periodically make changes for variety.

☐ **Check with the therapist**—the therapist will let you know if the sensory diet is adequately satisfying a child's needs.

The following list of possible activities is adapted from Kranowitz (1998, 2005) and the sources listed in the Further Reading section.

☐ **Alerting activities** for the *hyposensitive* child that seeks extra stimulation can include:

» eating crunchy foods

» drinking liquids of varying temperatures or with bubbles

» taking a shower

» jumping or bouncing.

☐ *Calming activities* to help the *hypersensitive* child decrease hyper-responsiveness to sensory stimulation might include:

» sucking on a hard candy, pacifier, frozen fruit, or ice cream bar

» back rubbing or hugging

» rocking or swaying slowly

» bathing.

☐ *Activities to develop tactile integration* could include:

» water painting: supply the child with water and a paintbrush and allow her to paint the sidewalk, or herself with imaginary paint

» finger drawing: with your finger, draw different letters or shapes on the child's back, and have her guess what you drew

» sandbox: hide small objects in a sandbox and have the child feel around for the objects without looking

» bath time: let the child experiment with different textures by having her rub soaps (shaving cream, lotion) and sponges (loofahs, washcloths, and plastic brushes) on her skin

» reading: encourage the child to read books (with or without you) in a rocking chair or bean bag

» pets: allow the child to stroke a cat, or brush a dog

» human sandwich: have the child lie face down on a gym mat; pretend to firmly rub mustard on the child with a sponge, paintbrush, or washcloth; then fold the mat over the child, and press firmly up and down to squish out the excess "mustard"; the child will enjoy the deep, soothing pressure of this activity

» dress up: set up a box with various textured clothing.

☐ *Activities to develop vestibular integration* might include:

» allowing the child to swing in a hammock

» navigating unstable surfaces: have the child walk on a beach, a grassy area, or a waterbed

» swinging: have her start on a swing where her feet touch the ground if she has a gravitational insecurity

» spinning: allow the child to swing on a merry-go-round or a tire swing; inside the child can use a swivel chair

» swimming, horseback riding, and bowling

» therapy ball: have the child try to balance on a large therapy ball.

☐ *Activities to develop proprioceptive integration* might include:

» housework: have the child carry grocery bags, laundry baskets, or a bunch of books; help the child push a vacuum cleaner; let the child help with digging or gardening

» pushing and pulling: let her push the stroller or a loaded wagon

» pillow crashing: have the child jump into, roll around, and burrow in a pile of pillows and cushions

» bear hugs: give tight, soothing hugs to your own child

» meal preparation

» playing catch: use a big ball or a pillow to play catch.

☐ *Activities to develop fine motor ("sensory motor") skills* might include:

  » practice sifting flour with a sifter

  » blocks and puzzles

  » arts and crafts (avoid choking hazards)

  » playdough.

Communication is key when it comes to increasing a child's success. Parents, classroom and other teachers, and school administrators must all be aware of a child's problems. However, try to be positive and brief. Avoid technical terms unless pressed for more specific information. Parents and teachers can share specific suggestions for the activities that work. For example, "My son is extremely sensitive to screeching noises. At home, he does best when we put cut up tennis balls under the chair legs to lessen the noise. Could you consider this in the classroom?"

Outcome

If a child has SID, the problems will probably lessen but continue as the child grows. She will learn to compensate for her difficulties, but there will still likely be some struggle as she performs everyday tasks. However, with the proper attention to the problem, a person can be given the opportunity to experience the world more smoothly.

CHAPTER 9

Tics and Tourette's

"That constant sniffling is driving me crazy! Some of the classmates find it so distracting, and a few are beginning to tease him about it. I know it's not his fault, but sometimes I feel tempted to ask him to stop. And why is he so nervous and always touching things?"

Basic definitions

What are tics?

Tics are rapid, repetitive actions that just happen to the child. They occur without any prolonged forethought by the person. Typically, tics tend to come and go, and change from one to another over time.

Tics are commonly classified into several types.

- *Simple motor tics.* "Motor" refers to the involvement of muscle movements. Common simple motor tics include simple movements such as eye blinks, nose scrunches, eyeball rolling, and neck thrusts.

- *Complex motor tics.* Complex motor tics involve movements that involve multiple groups of muscles. These might include body twisting, hopping, or shooting up of an arm.

- *Vocal tics.* These are tics that involve noises. Usually, the noise is a sniffling sound, throat clearing, squeak, bark, or echoing of what was just said. Only a small minority of patients with vocal tics actually have "coprolalia," which is the involuntary shouting of obscenities. Coprolalia should not be confused with simple cursing. Typical cursing is relevant to the current situation. In coprolalia, the taboo word occurs irrelevantly in the middle of a sentence. An example of coprolalia might be, "Could I please S-H-I-T have some maple syrup with my pancakes?" Sometimes, though, the coprolalia is just the blurting out of something socially totally inappropriate. For example, a person with a deformity might walk by and the result of coprolalia might be to shout out, "Freak!"

In addition, tics can be classified as either persistent (*chronic*) if they have occurred for at least a year, even if intermittently, or provisional (*transient*) if it has been less than one year since tic onset.

What is Tourette's syndrome?

Simply defined Tourette's criteria include:

- a combination of at least two motor tics and at least one vocal tic

- symptoms have lasted at least one year

- onset before 18 years old.

Tourette's is basically just a mixed vocal and motor tic disorder. That's all. I know parents who tell me, "I've gotten comfortable with John's noises and movements. Just don't tell me he has Tourette's." Tourette's is not degenerative. It is nothing to be afraid of. Most people who have Tourette's probably do not even know that they meet the criteria.

A complex problem

Having just simplified the definition of Tourette's, I must say that it is usually not nearly so simple.

Tourette's is a highly co-morbid condition. Dr. Leslie Packer, a psychologist specializing in Tourette's, calls it Tourette Syndrome "Plus," to indicate that so many people with Tourette's have other conditions such as obsessive-compulsive disorder (>80%) and anxiety (30%) (Harris and Wu 2010). Fully 60% of people with Tourette's have ADHD; conversely, 7% of people with ADHD have Tourette's (Waslick and Greenhill 2004, p.492). When looking specifically at 6–12-year-olds, Prince and Wilens (2009) found that 56% of those children who had tics (not necessarily full blown Tourette's) also had ADHD, and conversely, 27% of children with ADHD also had tics. Other frequently co-occurring conditions with tics include depression, learning disabilities, and autism spectrum disorder. Tourette's plays a major role in the syndrome mix. The associated problems may be at least as debilitating as the tics themselves.

Here are some medical facts (King and Leckman 2004, pp.709–715):

- Tics occur transiently in up to 18% of boys and 11% of girls.

- Tourette's syndrome occurs three to four times more often in boys than girls.

- A partial expression of Tourette's occurs in 1 out of 200 people.

- About 100,000 people in the US have the full Tourette's syndrome.

- If one identical twin has Tourette's, then the twin sibling has a more than 50% chance of having Tourette's. This appears to be a biological problem that then interacts with the environment to determine how strongly it will be expressed.

- OCD, anxiety, ADHD, and tics run strongly through the same families.

- Neuroanatomically, tics are due to a disorder in the planning loop between the cortex of the brain and deep-seated movement and sensory centers. This is a similar loop to that involved in OCD/anxiety.

- Biochemically, tics seem related to too much activity by the neurotransmitters dopamine and norepinephrine.

What about "nervous tics"?

Unless you already have the biological condition, stress does not cause tics. For people who are already prone to them, tics may be exacerbated by stressful situations, and, certainly, many people who have Tourette's have a co-occurring anxiety disorder. However, tics are not caused by stress. Let's get rid of that misconception right away.

A medical analogy to migraines may help the explanation. Stress may trigger migraines in a person who is prone to them, but it would be crazy to say to a person who is seeing flashing lights with a severe migraine headache, "Hey, why are you reacting so badly to the stress that your vision is affected?" Stress may be the exacerbating factor, but then the natural condition takes over.

Actually, sometimes tics are maximal when the child is totally comfortable—such as when the child is at home watching television with his parents. It is important for teachers and parents to realize all of this, or they may misinterpret themselves as having created a stressed-out child in a stressed environment.

The natural course of tics

The only constant feature of tics is that they are variable. They come for no apparent reason, hang around for different amounts of time, go away, come back, never come back, or come back as a different type. Fluctuation and change are the norms. Tics typically start between four to six years of age, and seem to become maximal around 10–12 years of age. By late teenage years, many children are significantly improved, and half or more are essentially tic-free.

Infections may worsen the tics, especially streptococcal infection (a condition called PANDAS: pediatric autoimmune neuropsychiatric disorders associated with strep).

Can people control their tics?

It is useless and counterproductive to ask a child to simply control his tics. It just does not work that way. After all, many people do not even know the tic is going to occur. It certainly is possible for some children to subconsciously suppress the tics temporarily (such as during the class play). Tics also tend to lessen when the child is engrossed in an activity, and during sleep. Some children learn to mask the tics by adding a more acceptable movement to the initial tic. For example, a sudden twitch of the arm may be masked by deliberately continuing the movement to brush the hair back.

However, without specific training, there is little long-term conscious control over tics, and the need to tic is irrepressible. It is like the need to breathe: a person can hold his breath for a while, but cannot do so indefinitely. So, can people exert control over their tics? Yes and no, but mostly no, unless explicitly taught how.

Treatment and accommodations

As we have seen, tics are very frequently accompanied by other conditions in the syndrome mix. Keep a look out for those difficulties, and learn about them in the appropriate chapters.

Understanding the child with tics

It is okay to notice the tics

Tics are typically not a problem as long as nobody gives the child a hard time about them. I'm not suggesting that family, friends, and teachers be too stupid to notice them—just that they do not make the child feel bad about them. No passing of judgment or teasing; just acceptance. Fortunately, most people get so used to the tics so that they no longer notice them—a process called habituation.

It is okay to have empathy for the tics

When a child is having a problem such as tics, it may be helpful to let the child know that you recognize and legitimize any difficulty he is experiencing. The child should know that someone is always available to talk about it, should he wish.

Dr. Packer has some "awareness exercises" on her website, which she suggests that caregivers try in order to understand what the child is going through (see the Further Reading section). For example, try to read a book while you twitch your head repetitively to the side every few seconds. Go ahead. Try it now while reading even one page. Distracting and annoying, isn't it? How would you like to live like that all day long? How would you like to go out in public while doing that?

So, empathy is good. Being available, when the child wants it, is good. However, bringing it to the child's constant attention certainly will not help, and is likely to be counterproductive.

It is not okay to bother the child about the tics

Peers may ask why a child does those movements. That is a legitimate question. The child with Tourette's might then respond, "My brain makes me do that." Or "It's an allergy." Or maybe even, "I have Tourette's, which causes tics… No, not Lyme disease tics, but funny movements called tics. I'm seeing a doctor about it. Thanks for asking." Typically, the peer responds, "Okay, throw the ball!" That type of interchange is excellent. At times, though, peers tease the child. That is not acceptable.

In the classroom
Educating classmates

In some cases, the parents or teacher may need to briefly educate the students about tics with an open discussion. It is harder to tease a child about something he already "admits" to. I've known some children who start the year with a presentation to the class about Tourette's. Be sure to discuss any public discussion of the problem with the child and the parents first. Dr. Leslie Packer gives some detailed pointers on such a presentation at her "Tourette Syndrome Plus" website (see the Further Reading section).

Teasing may not be the only problem

In general, then, tics are only a problem when other people make them so. There are, however, some kids for whom the tics will still be problematic.

- For some children, just the presence of the tics affects their self-image, even if no one else is giving them a hard time.

- Sometimes, tics interfere with daily activities. For example, constant neck or eye jerks may interfere with reading or cause neck pain. A constant cough may disrupt the child and the whole class.

- Sometimes the movements affect handwriting and/or reading.

- Some children expend so much mental energy on the tics (either from trying to suppress them or from dealing with the embarrassment) that they may appear inattentive.

Specific classroom accommodations

Some of Dr. Packer's suggestions for accommodations for children with tics include the following:

☐ *The teacher should model acceptance of the tics.* If the teacher reacts negatively to them, what do we expect the students to do?

☐ *Allow the child to leave the room* if the tics become overwhelming. This may be especially important in quiet settings such as the library, study hall, or assemblies.

☐ *Do not ask the child to leave the room.* That appears punitive for something over which the child has no control.

☐ *Provide extra time* if the tics slow down the work.

☐ *Provide creative accommodations* for difficulties. As an example, if reading aloud is embarrassing, consider avoiding it. If tics interfere with writing; then use oral tests, a scribe, or a computer.

☐ *Provide extra supervision if the child is being teased* in situations such as recess or lunch.

☐ *Allow preferential seating.* Some children with tics prefer to sit in the back of the class so that no one can see the tics.

For most children with moderate tics, life will be okay with simple education, understanding, and reassurance about the condition. When the tics remain a significant problem in a child's life, then we may need to go to more specific treatments—the choices being Habit Reversal Training (HRT), or the more complete Comprehensive Behavioral Intervention for Tics (CBIT)—and/or medication.

Habit Reversal Training (HRT) and Comprehensive Behavioral Intervention for Tics (CBIT)

If you are fortunate enough to have a motivated child and an available therapist trained in the technique of HRT or CBIT, these therapies are typically first line. They teach lifelong skills, and are essentially risk- and medication-free.

In HRT:

• the patient is trained to recognize the glimmer of a premonition that precedes the tic

• the patient is then trained to perform some competing response that makes it physically impossible to perform the tic. For example, if the child senses that he is about to have an inhaling sniff tic, he exhales instead. This breaks the cycle of premonition that will obligatorily lead to fulfillment of the tic. With a course of weekly sessions over a few months, the premonitions and the tics diminish.

A full program, such as CBIT, adds education about Tourette's, relaxation techniques, and an individualized approach to changing daily life factors that make tics worse. It works for many people. In one study in the Journal of the American Medical Association (Piacentini 2010), significant symptom improvement was achieved in 52.5% of the children who underwent CBIT versus just 18.5% of children receiving the control treatment.

Medication for tics

If none of the above is effective enough (or not available), medication may be an option. Medications do not cure the symptoms; they just control them for the days that the child takes them. Put another way, current practice works on the premise that there is no long-term medical harm if we hold off on medication. We will not have to kick ourselves and say, "Oh, if we had only started medication earlier." Starting earlier would have had no effect on the tics today.

The critical questions, then, as to starting medication are as follows:

- Is the issue a quirk or a problem? It is a problem when the tics diminish the child's self-esteem or function.

- Is the problem worth the possible side effects of medication for this child, at this point in time?

The commonly used medications to treat tic disorders are as follows:

- Catapres (clonidine) or Tenex (guanfacine) are frequently the mediations tried first. They may help the tics, and may help any co-occurring ADHD (particularly the impulsive part). The most common side effects can be sedation, and lowered blood pressure and pulse.

- Risperdal (risperidone) and other "neuroleptics" are usually quite effective for tics, and may help control angry or aggressive behaviors as well. They do not help inattention. Common side effects include sedation, metabolic changes, and weight gain. There are also rare, potentially serious, side effects.

Note that the stimulants used to treat ADHD have been felt by many doctors to at times alter the frequency of the tics, although recent research does not tend to support those impressions. See Chapter 14 for more information on the medical treatment of tic disorders.

CHAPTER 10

Depression

"I just don't know what has happened to Jane. She has so little energy! That twinkle in her eye is gone. Nothing seems to motivate or excite her anymore. Sometimes she can be so irritable, and yells at me over nothing. Sometimes, she curls up in a ball and can't get up. Then she can't fall asleep at night, or wake up in the morning. She's always late. Her eating habits are all off, too. We thought it might be mono or Lyme, but her tests just came back negative.

"She tries to put on a brave face at school, but her grades are slipping. Her absences from school make it worse—she can't possibly catch up. She won't go in for extra help. 'Why should I? Nothing interests me. Nothing seems to matter or be any fun,' she says."

Defining depression and dysthymia

In DSM-5, the American Psychiatric Association (2013) makes the distinction between a major depressive episode (which is a severe, typically episodic illness representing a clear-cut change from baseline); versus dysthymia (which is a more smoldering condition); versus disruptive mood dysregulation disorder (which is chronic irritability/anger with frequent explosions). Here's a little more detail on each condition.

- *A major depressive episode* is marked by the experience, for most of the hours of every day for at least two weeks, of:

  ○ feelings of depressed mood (sadness, emptiness, hopelessness, or loss of "zest") and/or

  ○ daily activities no longer hold any appeal or produce any pleasure.

  There may be feelings of worthlessness or guilt, and recurrent thoughts of death may occur. The ability to concentrate or make decisions may be altered. Before adulthood, this may all manifest simply as irritability. In addition, there are physical symptoms of depression, including sleep problems, fatigue, restlessness, loss of energy, weight gain, or unintentional weight loss. All of these problems must cause actual dysfunction in a person's life for at least two weeks in order to make a diagnosis of a major depressive episode (APA 2013).

- *A persistent depressive disorder (dysthymia)* to use DSM-5 terminology, is defined as depression for most of the day, for more days than not, over a two-year period (or a one-year period of irritability for children/adolescents). There may be physical symptoms as seen in a major depressive episode. Over this period, the symptoms never resolve for more than two months, and cause functional impairment in the person's life (APA 2013).

- *Disruptive mood dysregulation disorder (DMDD)* is a newly coined category of DSM-5, marked by a chronic mood of severe irritability or anger that is persistent (i.e., for most of the day, most days, for at least one year). There are also severe temper outbursts occurring at least three times per week. These are not just regular tantrums, they must occur in at least two settings (such as at home, at school, or with friends), be developmentally inappropriate for age, and be out of proportion to the trigger, and may be verbal (such as verbal rages) or physical aggression towards people or things. This is a new diagnostic category designed to prevent possible overdiagnosis of bipolar disorder in children currently in the age range of 7–18 years old (APA 2013, p.155). It turns out that the *chronically* irritable, explosive kids described in this disorder are at risk of future depression and/or anxiety disorder, but have a very low rate of becoming bipolar disorder. According to DSM-5, bipolar is marked by truly *episodic* spells of altered mood and behavior (which are well distinguished from the child's typical behavior). DMDD also lacks the defined spells of mania with its elevated mood and grandiose thoughts of bipolar. Hence, disruptive mood dysregulation disorder is included here under the chapter heading "depression" rather than the chapter on "bipolar disorder." The condition entitled "intermittent explosive disorder" may also be considered in the differential diagnosis; it does not involve persistent alteration of mood in between the outbursts. See Table 10.1 for a summary of conditions most notable for mood and/or explosive behaviors. ADHD, anxiety, depression, autism spectrum, and oppositional defiant disorders must also be considered in the differential.

Mood disorders can appear differently through the lifespan. Younger children may be unable to verbalize their sadness. Instead, the only symptoms that caregivers may notice are irritability, getting into fights, or avoidance. Alternatively, they may present with physical symptoms such as headaches or abdominal pain. Older children and adolescents may present with the more typical core symptoms of sadness and emptiness along with loss of motivation, pleasure, energy, and self-esteem.

TABLE 10.1: Classification of mood and/or explosive behaviors in DSM-5

Condition	Course of mood	Explosive behaviors
Major depressive episode	*Episodic* depression (for at least two weeks)	Not a defining feature, but explosions may occur during depressive episodes
Bipolar I disorder	*Episodic* mania (for at least seven days) +/− depression (for at least two weeks)	Not a defining feature but explosions may occur during episodes of mania or depression
Bipolar II disorder	*Episodic* hypomania (for at least four days) + depression (for at least two weeks)	Not a defining feature but explosions may occur during episodes of hypomania or depression
Persistent depressive disorder (dysthymia)	*Chronic* depression (measured in years)	Not a defining feature
Disruptive mood dysregulation disorder	*Chronic* severe irritability (for at least one year)	Defining feature (at least three times per week)
Intermittent explosive disorder	*Normal* mood	Defining feature

Real-life symptoms

Depression in children is easy to miss. Children under age seven, in particular, may be unable to directly state their sadness. Thus, we need to keep an eye out for an expanded range of symptoms.

- *Sadness*—"Mommy, I hate feeling so down! I just feel so empty and hopeless. I've really got a pretty good life. Why do I feel this way?"

- *Feeling of emptiness*—"I just feel so, so, so alone."

- *Self-esteem problems*—"I'm just no good at anything! I'm so stupid!"

- *Withdrawal/loss of interests*—the mother bemoans about her child, "Sleep. Do nothing. Sleep. I can't get him to do anything except just hang around. He no longer wants to do anything, and when he does get out, he doesn't get any pleasure from it."

- *Irritability*—"Jane just walks around with a chip on her shoulder. For no reason, she's just always in a lousy mood. My son John—the one with ADHD—is usually happy as a clam as long as I leave him alone. He snaps at me when I make a demand on him like coming to dinner. My depressed child, though, just walks around looking miserable. She snaps at me even if I leave her alone."

- *Bodily complaints*—"Jane is always complaining about headaches, or maybe her stomach is hurting her. I've been to lots of doctors. We've had MRIs (magnetic resonance imaging) and blood tests. They tell me it is just stress."

- *Sleep problems*—"Jane can't seem to fall asleep. She is always worrying about something. Sometimes, she naps all afternoon. We can't get her up in the morning, so she's always late for school."

- *Appetite problems*—"She keeps eating and is getting fatter. No wonder she is so depressed!" The last thing that a teenager with depression needs is the additional problem with self-image that comes from being overweight. Loss of weight can also accompany depression.

- *Concentration problems*—"I don't get it. She never had trouble concentrating before." If concentration problems suddenly begin in the later school years, we need to be suspicious about diagnosing ADHD. New onset attention problems suggest another issue, such as depression, anxiety, drug use, etc.

- *Stress on the family*—"I can't bear to see my child like this!" First, the child's lack of effort—along with his irritability—is exceptionally hard to live with. Even more difficult, though, is watching your child be unhappy. What could be worse?

- *Stress on the teacher*—"I went into teaching to get kids excited about this subject. But I can't seem to get this kid involved. I offer her help, but she never takes it. She doesn't even seem to try." What could be worse for a teacher than to have a student who is unable to muster any motivation?

- *Thoughts of death*—the horrific truth is that suicide is a prominent cause of death in adolescents. We all need to be vigilant, and take any talk of self-harm seriously.

Suicide

Suicide is the third leading cause of death for teenagers, and is an ever-present concern in depression. Complete evaluation of a child's risk for suicide needs individualized, professional input—and is difficult even then. Full discussion of suicide is beyond the scope of this text.

Some of the major risk factors for suicide are:

- a previous history of suicide attempts or threats (although most completed suicides are not preceded by "unsuccessful" attempts)

- previous attempts that have utilized techniques other than ingestion or superficial cutting

- a history of non-suicidal self-harm (such as cutting)

- the presence of a plan for suicide

- ongoing wishes to die

- thoughts of suicide

- feelings of depression, hopelessness, anxiety, and/or isolation

- agitation, irritability, delusional, or other psychosis

- a stressful event (such as loss of parent, school problem, or romantic break-up)

- being exposed to others' suicidal behavior

- being male (especially 16–19 years of age) versus female

- sexual orientation as gay/lesbian/bisexual

- alcohol or drug abuse in patient or his family

- impulsive behavior

- aggressive behavior in males, and panic attacks in females

- a history of bullying

- having bipolar disorder

- a family history of attempted/completed suicide, bipolar or childhood maltreatment

- cultural or religious views about suicide

- lack of access or use of available help.

(AACAP 2012; CDC 2012)

Get the guns and dangerous medicines out of the house

According to the Centers for Disease Control (CDC)'s latest data derived from the National Vital Statistics Report (Murphy 2013), of the roughly 30,000 gun-related deaths in the US during 2010, about 20,000 of them were due to suicide (with most of the remaining third of cases being homicides). There were 600 unintentional deaths from firearms. Since many suicide attempts occur within one hour of a spike in suicidal feelings, ready access to a lethal means such as a gun is a recipe for disaster. It turns out that 85% of attempted suicides with guns are fatal, whereas suicide attempts with pills are fatal only 2% of the time (Tavernise 2013). With guns, you don't typically get a second chance. If that weren't enough to dissuade parents from having a gun accessible in the house, how about this, "An analysis of 400 firearms deaths that occurred in the home, showed that, for every self-defense homicide in the home, there were nearly five times as many domestic criminal homicides and 37 suicides" (Brent *et al.* 2013).

Block access to guns and dangerous drugs—get them out of the house, especially if concerned about suicide in a family member. If that is not an option, then at least be sure to have dangerous medications secured, and any guns and ammunition inaccessible and locked safely apart.

If you have concerns about suicide, restrict access to harmful situations, do not leave the person alone, and immediately contact your doctor and/or go to the emergency room and/or call 911 in the US.

Neurobiology of depression

Like many behavioral problems, depression is often a combination of environmental effects on a predisposed brain. One marker that this emotion is due to a biological illness (rather than just being "weak in spirit") is that biologically depressed children often know that their feelings of sadness don't make sense. Their feeling of sadness feels unwelcome, unacceptable, and imposed upon them. Sometimes, though, the depressed child does lose objective reality and truly feels that her life is actually horrible. Of course, sometimes, the life she is living *is* truly horrible.

On a biochemical level, depression seems due to a largely genetic dysfunction of the right parietal-temporal cortex stemming from:

- too little of the neurotransmitter norepinephrine released by nerves in the locus coeruleus (part of the brainstem) onto the cortex, and

- too little of the neurotransmitter serotonin released by the median raphe (also part of the brainstem) onto the cortex.

The role of certain hormones is also being investigated.

Treatment

Counseling

Cognitive behavioral therapy (CBT) is typically part of the treatment. In order for therapy to even be successfully started, though, it helps when the child:

- recognizes that there *is* a painful problem; otherwise, what is there to talk about?

- recognizes that he has a role in that problem; otherwise, why should he see the therapist? If—in the child's mind—the parent or teacher is the one with the problem, then *they* should be having the counseling! See Chapter 7 on anxiety/OCD for a description of CBT.

Medication

Given the biochemical underpinning commonly involved with depression, it makes sense that medication often plays a key role in treatment.

The mainstay of antidepressants is a class of medication called the selective serotonin reuptake inhibitors (SSRIs). These medicines inhibit the removal of serotonin from the synapse, leading to raised serotonin levels. Roughly, a half to two-thirds of children have a significant beneficial effect from the SSRIs. The medications may take one or two months to take hold. If one SSRI does not work or is not tolerated, another one may be tried. Note that the SSRIs can worsen bipolar disorder, and may have other side effects as described in Chapter 14 on medications. Although other SSRIs are often used in common practice, only Prozac (fluoxetine) actually has current US Food and Drug Administration approval for use in children with depression who are eight years and older, and Lexapro (escitalopram) for children who are 12 years and older.

Before the introduction of the SSRIs, the mainstay of treatment had been the tricyclic antidepressants such as Elavil, Tofranil, or Pamelor. Multiple controlled studies have shown that the tricyclics do not work in childhood depression. They are not considered a first-line treatment. Emerging evidence points to a potential role for omega-3 fatty acids in the treatment of mood disorders (Strawn *et al.* 2013).

These and the other medications are discussed in Chapter 14.

Overall, it may take months to find the correct dose of the correct medication, and even then, medication may not help.

Combined CBT and medication treatment

The following conclusions are derived from a randomized control study on adolescent depression sponsored by the National Institute of Mental Health (March and Vitiello 2009).

- Combined CBT and medication works significantly faster than does either therapy alone.

- CBT helps to minimize the increased risk of suicidality brought about by medication.

- Thus, combined CBT and medication should typically be the treatments of choice for moderate to severe depression.

- In order to consolidate gains in most moderately to severely ill adolescents, six to nine months of therapy are required.

- CBT may be sufficient by itself in mild cases of depression, particularly where there are no suicidal issues in socio-demographically advantaged children.

Adjusting the school environment

Parents also need to bring the school in as part of the team. Unfortunately, there is frequently such a stigma and concern about privacy attached to "psychiatric disorders" that no one tells the teachers about the problem. Left in the dark, the teacher often feels no recourse other than to either come down hard on the child or give up on her. But there is much that can be done to help at school. The school's psychology/guidance counselors/ special education staff can help.

☐ *Teachers need to allow time to make up for missed work.* Children with depression often miss a lot of school. Don't expect the child to seek out the extra help himself. He's depressed.

☐ *Don't consider the lack of effort to be a deliberate choice.* Loss of motivation is a cardinal symptom of depression.

☐ *Try to avoid the vicious cycle of depression → school failure → more depression.* We don't want to let academic problems exacerbate the underlying depression.

☐ *Accommodate poor attention span during depressive state.* (See Chapter 3 on ADHD.)

☐ *Children with depression may be physiologically unable to get up in the morning.* Such medically related tardiness will need to be excused, and the school schedule adjusted to fit the child's needs.

☐ *Consider school issues that may have triggered depression in the first place.* In particular, it is not uncommon for bright, cute, inattentive girls with ADHD to go undiagnosed until high school. After so many years of being told that they could do better, things finally fall apart and depression sets in. Always be vigilant for one condition in the syndrome mix causing, mimicking, or exacerbating the symptoms of another condition.

☐ *Talk of suicide should be taken seriously.* School guidance counselors, parents, and therapists should be notified immediately.

Outcome

Depression is extremely common. At any given time, some 1–4% of children will be experiencing major depression, and overall, some 15–20% of kids will have a major depressive episode before becoming an adult (Weller, Weller and Danielyan 2004). That is a lot of children. That probably means the average teacher has taught lots of depressed students, without knowing it.

The good news is that some 90% of children with depression will go into remission within a year. The bad news is that up to a half will have a relapse (Weller *et al.* 2004).

Depression is an incredibly terrible, empty feeling. It is horrible. It needs to evoke from us an incredibly empathic response.

CHAPTER 11

Bipolar Disorder

"I'm really scared... It's like he's possessed. Most weeks, he is the sweetest, kindest person. He would do anything for you. Then, for no reason, something sweeps over his brain and he turns on me. There's screaming and yelling and things flying around the room. Once he gets going, his rages may take hours. He can be irritable and moody for days on end. Sometimes, he's so down that I'm afraid for his own safety—not to mention my own. Sometimes, though, he's so 'up' that his judgment gets really poor. He spends all day and night buying things! Often, though, it always seems to be worse when he's at home. When I tell people about it, they look at me like I'm crazy. My father-in-law was manic-depressive, and it led him to a drinking problem. I'm so scared..."

"Manic depression" and "bipolar depression" are the old names. "Bipolar Disorder" (BD) is the scientific name in DSM-5, which removes the word *depression*—since the criteria for only certain types of bipolar disorder actually mandate depression as part of the disorder. Call it what you will, it can be a horror. The intermittent mood changes that take the brain hostage—either up or down—are frightening, confusing, and often dangerous. To make matters worse, people with BD are at a hugely high risk for co-morbid conditions of the syndrome mix.

What is bipolar disorder?

There are actually two major forms of bipolar disorder (BD): bipolar I disorder and bipolar II disorder. In order to understand the bipolar disorders and describe their difference, we first need to have a handle on the terms "manic episode," "hypomanic episode," and "major depressive episode" as described by DSM-5 (although controversy still exists about the criteria for these conditions). *Note the use of the word "episode" in each of these terms—an indication of the importance in DSM-5 of these spells being episodic, i.e., they represent both (a) distinct time periods of (b) distinct behaviors that are clearly distinguishable from the person's baseline.*

Manic episode

Manic episodes are distinct periods of at least seven days duration (which differ from the person's baseline behavior) marked by:

- mood that is elevated, grandiose, euphoric, or irritable, and

- increased energy and/or goal-directed behavior.

During these episodes, there needs to be *marked dysfunctioning* and at least three of the following symptoms (four symptoms if the mood is only irritable).

- Exaggerated self-esteem or grandiose thinking.

- Lack of need for sleep (to be distinguished from insomnia, which is trouble falling into or maintaining sleep).

- Excessively talkative.

- Racing or flighty speech.

- Easily distracted by irrelevant stimuli.

- Extreme goal-directed behavior.

- Extreme involvement in behavior that may have negative outcomes. In children, this may manifest as concocting multiple, elaborate yet unrealistic projects.

Hypomanic episode

Hypomanic episodes meet the above criteria for manic episodes, except that they:

- only need to last at least four days of distinct behaviors (versus seven days for manic spell), and

- do *not* cause significant functional impairment.

In fact, because they do not cause significant harm, they are frequently not brought to the doctor's attention.

Major depressive episode

Major depressive episodes are described in Chapter 10 on depression. *Twelve percent of bipolar II patients are originally diagnosed with major depressive disorder* before a hypomanic episode is diagnosed (APA 2013, p.136). This is an important issue since the medical treatments are hugely different, and standard antidepressants such as Prozac (fluoxetine) can provoke mania. For more information see Chapter 14 on medication.

Defining the bipolar disorders in DSM-5

With these terms under our belt, we can quickly put the building blocks together to define the two patterns of bipolar disorder.

- *Bipolar I must have at least one manic episode.* That's it. It may (and frequently does) or may not also have episodes of major depression or hypomania. One manic spell as above and you're bipolar I for the rest of your life. Thus, note that a person can be "bipolar" while exhibiting only one of the "poles," i.e., mania.

- *Bipolar II must have at least one hypomanic episode and at least one major depressive episode.* That's all it can have. If there's a full manic spell, then we're back to bipolar I. Apparently, these distinctions make sense scientifically. Note that bipolar II is not necessarily less severe than bipolar I.

That's how DSM-5 sees bipolar disorder. I must point out that many doctors feel that the episodic requirement of the criteria may apply to adults, but does not necessarily apply to children. These doctors view bipolar children as frequently having chronic, persistent extreme irritability as well as possible ultra-rapid cycling in and out of manic and/or depressive states (including up to several times per day, or even simultaneously), perhaps with resultant severe rages (see Papolos 2006, for example). DSM-5 explicitly dismisses this view of chronicity, and thus carefully constructed the DSM-5 criteria above of clearly distinct episodes that differ from the child's baseline. In addition, DSM-5 created the diagnostic condition of "Disruptive Mood Dysregulation Disorder" under the category of Depressive Disorders as a place to put chronically irritable, raging children without labeling them as bipolar or considering them to be "pre-bipolar." The authors of DSM-5 state that "nonepisodic irritability in youth is associated with an elevated risk for anxiety disorders and major depressive disorder, but not bipolar disorder" (APA 2013, p.137).

Additional features of bipolar

- *Failure to perceive manic spells as requiring help.* In fact, some find that the spells help their creativity, yet fail to see the social and even legal consequences of their impaired judgment.

- *Highly increased suicide risk*—felt to be at least 15 times higher than control. (Bipolar II is at a higher risk than bipolar I.)

- *Highly genetic*—with a ten fold higher risk if you have a relative with bipolar. (The closer genetically related, the higher the risk.)

- *Extremely high incidence of alcohol or other substance abuse.*

- *May become hostile to others—"go for the jugular."*

- *High incidence of co-morbidity, including:*
  - anxiety disorder in ¾ of bipolar I patients
  - ADHD in over ½ of bipolar I patients
  - 60% of bipolar II patients have three or more co-morbidities.

- *May have extreme rages that may last for hours.*

- *Papolos (2006) notes the following common features of childhood BD:* extreme sensitivity to stimuli, extreme sexuality, extreme craving for sweets, extreme separation anxiety, extreme fear of death, and extreme heat sensitivity.

- *Notice how often the word "extreme" is used* in this disorder of distinct "poles."

- *Nightmares and night terrors.*

- *Often, lack of need for sleep.*

- *Some people with BD have hallucinations.*

- *Typically, most of the child's symptoms are shown primarily at home*—as if the parents did not feel bad enough already. Parents may be surprised to hear that their child is a little angel at school; teachers may be surprised to hear that the child is so difficult at home.

Read *The Bipolar Child* by Dimitri Papolos for more details (see the Further Reading section).

Confusion with other conditions

Once again, conditions can co-occur, or can be confused with or exacerbate each other. As above, a host of neuropsychiatric conditions turn out to be associated with BD. Keeping the provisos above in mind, consider BD rather than ADHD (or in addition to ADHD) when there are the above symptoms or:

- a family history of bipolar disorder, substance abuse, or suicide

- prolonged temper outbursts and mood swings (in BD, the angry, violent, sadistic, and disorganized outbursts can last for hours, versus typically fewer than 30 minutes in ADHD)

- bipolar rages arising typically from parental limit setting (versus ADHD rages, which are usually from over-stimulation)

- walking around with an angry "chip on your shoulder" (BD people often walk around looking miserable for no apparent reason. In ADHD, the kids are typically quite chipper up until the moment that someone/something frustrates or overwhelms them. To put it another way, depressed people are irritable for days or weeks on end; ADHD people are easily irritated)

- oppositional and defiant behaviors

- "intentionally" aggressive, explosive, or risk-seeking behaviors

- symptoms that worsen with stimulants (such as Ritalin) or antidepressants

- morning irritability that may last hours in BD (versus minutes in ADHD)

- separation anxiety, bad dreams, disturbed sleep, or fascination with gore

- you never know what child you are going to get this week.

The distinction of bipolar versus disruptive mood dysregulation disorder has already been covered in Table 10.1 above, and is based primarily of the episodic nature of bipolar. Consider "intermittent explosive disorder" when there are, well, intermittent explosions but no mood issues. (See Chapter 12 on oppositional defiant disorder.)

Treatment

First, follow the suggestions in Chapter 2 on the general principles of treatment. All of the suggestions apply particularly to bipolar. Go ahead... Re-read that chapter... We'll still be right here. [Queue noise of finger tapping while we wait for the reader to return.]

In the classroom

Bipolar is *overwhelming*. The key is to "underwhelm" by keeping it predictable, calm, and secure. Can you imagine what it must be like to have unexpected, monsoon-sized, tidal waves of inexplicable emotion sweep over you? These children need a reliable, soothing environment. Many of these suggestions could be used by good teachers for all students.

☐ *Make routines predictable.* Let everyone (child and parents) know about weekly assignments such as spelling tests. Consider keeping a schedule of the day's events on the blackboard.

☐ *Give adequate notification before making transitions.* Make sure that the child actually hears and processes these warnings—he may be preoccupied.

☐ *Give extra time for transitions.* Allow him to finish a task before moving on. Failure to do so may prove extremely frustrating, and the precipitation of a meltdown does not help anyone.

☐ *Allow plenty of breaks*, both planned and as needed.

☐ *Arrange "secret" hand codes* that the student can give to the teacher to indicate present or impending moods (e.g., thumb up means "good," five outstretched fingers means "stressed," etc.).

☐ *Allow—and encourage use of—a minute to reflect* before the child makes his choice.

☐ *Allow the child to pull back* when he feels overwhelmed—with no hassling questions. Let the child go to the bathroom, for a drink of water, or to a pre-selected place or person that functions as a safe haven. These types of pop-off valve activities should be arranged in advance of their need. School safety policies need to be considered.

☐ *If classroom commotion* is a de-stabilizing force for the child:

» have the child sit preferentially in a quiet part of the room

» have the child sit next to calm, quiet students.

☐ *Some students may not tolerate lunchroom or recess noise.* They may need an aide at those times, or to spend those periods elsewhere.

☐ *Avoid direct confrontation!* (See Rule 2 in Chapter 2.) If certain activities trigger meltdowns, then try to steer clear of them. For example, if a child screams before going to music class (maybe he has a sensory integration problem?) then don't take him there. A useful tactic is to offer a child two acceptable alternatives to choose from.

☐ *Some bipolar kids need an aide.* It's hard to stop class and publicly come over to a child who is "losing it." An extra aide in the class can quietly come over and intervene while the main teacher goes on with the lesson. Sometimes, the child will need her own aide—although some older children, in particular, will not tolerate that. Other children might be candidates for an "inclusion" class, in which case several special needs children share an aide or special education teacher in a class of otherwise "typical" children. Hopefully, the extra helpers will have some training in dealing with the particular set of problems faced by the child.

☐ *Bipolar children also need lots of positive support!*

☐ *Say something nice* every five minutes. Say 12 nice things for every negative comment. Find *something* nice to say, even if it's just saying, "Billy, I like the way you merely yelled at Tommy, rather than bopping him on the head."

☐ *Teach other students to accept diversity.* Teach peers how different brains can learn and react differently.

Remember, too, that punishing a bipolar child for a rage attack makes as much sense as punishing a child who has epilepsy for having a seizure. Do not punish children for behavior that is out of their control. It is neither fair nor useful. And, again, federal law in the US prohibits punishing children for their disability.

A child's *rapport with a teacher* can make or break a school year. Teacher traits that are beneficial to the special needs child include:

- flexibility (do not get involved in power struggles. Give *palatable* alternatives. Threats and ultimatums can set off the child into making poor choices)

- patience

- sense of humor

- being receptive to suggestions from others.

- being structured with a sense of humor.

Don't *underestimate* your role in a child's success, and don't necessarily *overestimate* your role in a child's failures.

Communication between school and parents

Caregivers should share amongst themselves:

- what strategies work, and just as importantly, what strategies don't work

- what is happening in their sphere, because it may spill over into the rest of the child's life

- what academic areas need more work, and which are causing stress or taking too much time

- what times of day make the most sense for particular activities—during the course of the day, there are likely to be variations in a child's attention, frustration tolerance, or medication effects.

Feedback about medication effects is essential. Teachers and parents are the eyes and ears for the physician. Doctors completely depend on the feedback that they receive. We cannot judge a medication's "real-world" effectiveness while the child is in the office. Giving feedback is not a presumptuous imposition; it is essential. When presented in a helpful manner, such feedback is usually well taken by everyone. Doctors need to know the following things:

- Does the medicine work?

- Does the medicine's effectiveness have peaks and valleys?

- Are there side effects, such as sleepiness, agitation, or increased appetite?

- Does the child need allowance for extra snacks or water breaks?

Caregivers should communicate *directly* with each other. Many children with BD may not be accurate historians as they relate their trials and tribulations between parents and teachers—especially those kids who also have oppositional defiant disorder (ODD).

- Direct communication eliminates the unreliable middleman.

- Use a phone, email, or a journal that goes back and forth with the child's backpack.

Dealing with manic spells

The life of a child with BD is plagued by mood swings. No one— not the child, the parent, nor the teacher—knows what kind of kid is going to show up today. Some days, the child will be manic, with either expansive energy or irritability. Suggestions for handling such behavior include the following strategies:

- Allow the children physical outlets for their driven energy. Let them be the ones to hand out and pick up paper, wash the board, or to deliver the attendance list to the office. Allow them to get up and use the computer.

- Direct them to productive hands-on projects.

- Help them set realistic goals, with reasonably sized projects.

Dealing with depressive spells

- See Chapter 10 on depression.

- Let them know you understand.

- Allow medically related morning tardiness. Depressed children may have physiological trouble waking up in the morning.

- Talk of suicide should be taken seriously. Parents and therapists should be notified expediently.

- Accommodate their poor attention during mood swings.

Classify the child as "Otherwise Health Impaired"

"Otherwise Health Impaired" (OHI) is the most appropriate special education category for BD students. This categorization validates that bipolar is a true medical health condition. Unfortunately, the alternative classification is "emotional disability" (ED). ED seems to imply that the child's behavioral problems are "emotional," i.e., that they somehow are due to poor upbringing and never bothering to learn basic appropriate behavior—a clearly counterproductive model. BD children may also merit other classifying labels, such as learning disabled, ADHD, and ODD.

Addressing specific problems

Deal with typically associated learning problems. Many children with BD have problems in the areas of:

- attention

- organization and analysis of learned material

- problem-solving skills

- memory and recall of learned material

- medication side effects, such as sedation or even mild cognitive slowing.

Address problems in social interactions. BD kids may have problems with social interactions that may benefit from:

- social skills classes

- rehearsal of appropriate responses in advance of typical problems (set up mock stories and act/write out productive responses. Discuss "what if" scenarios)

- private discussion about inappropriate responses after the problem occurs.

Accommodate associated attention deficits. Children with bipolar disorder are at extremely high risk for having co-occurring ADHD as well (Weller *et al.* 2004). Even without ADHD as an additional primary diagnosis, the child's attention span may worsen during manic or depressive episodes. See Chapter 3 on ADHD, and consider doing the following things:

- Decrease the workload (e.g., do four out of five problems). Focus on quality rather than quantity.

- Give extra time for tests and schoolwork.

- Check in on their progress frequently, and give positive prompts.

- Have them sit near the teacher.

- Avoid excessive classroom heat or dim lights that may interfere with attention.

Medication

The complicated issue of treating bipolar disorder is addressed in Chapter 14 on medication. Along with therapeutic counseling, in general, medications will be an integral part of the treatment. Sometimes, though, their side effects can be significant.

CHAPTER 12

Oppositional Defiant Disorder (ODD) and Intermittent Explosive Disorder

A four-year-old boy was told by his nursery school teacher that he had to lie down on his cot at rest-time. The boy said that he was not going to lie down. The teacher insisted upon compliance. The boy calmly walked over the cot, urinated on it, and announced, "I guess that I don't have to lie down on it, now." This true story was the harbinger of future oppositional behaviors.

What is oppositional defiant disorder?

This is an unpleasant chapter. Throughout the rest of the book, it is fairly easy to take the child's side—at least during a calm moment. Oppositional defiant disorder (ODD) may commonly have a biological underpinning, but the behaviors seen in this condition test the limits of our ability to exercise sympathy. As Barkley (2013, p.5) has pointed out, the kids who need our help the most may ask for it in the most unloving way.

The symptoms of ODD according to DSM-5 include: often losing temper or being easily annoyed; and arguing with authority figures. There are many kids in the syndrome mix who meet those criteria when the demands placed upon them exceed their skill set. (Remember Ross Greene's dictum (2010): children already do well when they can.) To me, though, the defining and unique features of ODD are the following additional possible DSM-5 symptoms: resentful, deliberately annoying, actively defies, spiteful, vindictive, and blaming others. Typically, the children with ODD don't see themselves as being the cause of the problems, justifying their behavior as a response to their circumstances or demands being placed upon them.

In general, I find the term *oppositional defiant disorder* to be potentially counterproductive and harmful. By viewing the children as "deliberately annoying" or "spiteful," it sets the stage for a power struggle, with the adult likely to come down heavily on the child—"I'll show him who's boss!" While there *are* some non-negotiable rules, this is typically the wrong approach. These kids already are overwhelmed. They need to be defused, not further inflamed. A better approach is to stay calm and figure out what is triggering the negative behavior. Often, the negative behavior is not truly volitional and deliberate. As an illustration, I doubt that any child with a normally functioning brain, growing up in a normal environment, ever had the following debate with himself upon awakening, "Gee, it's a new day. I could either comply with the rules, get As, get hugs and kisses and praise; *or*, I could annoy everyone, feel irritable, get bad grades, and be punished. Boy, the second choice sounds so good! I'm going to go for it!" (If they did choose the second option, I would posit that the child either didn't have a normally functioning brain or a normal environment.)

It's not that there aren't kids who meet the criteria for ODD—there are lots of them. It's just that I prefer to think first of oppositional defiant behaviors as frequently being symptoms of some other problem that we have not solved yet. Indeed, ODD is rarely seen in isolation. Often, the negative behaviors tend to improve with the treatment of the underlying problem(s). One way or another, it is crucial to address the symptoms of ODD, since children with such symptoms are at higher risk of developing more severe and dangerous disruptive behaviors.

Types of disruptive behavioral disorders

ODD is the least severe of the three types of disruptive behavioral disorders. Full definitions can be found in the DSM-5.

- *Oppositional defiant disorder (ODD).* ODD children appear unwilling to conform (even with an intriguing task). They may be negative, deliberately annoying, argumentative, angry, and spiteful. They often seem to get a "charge" out of giving other people a hard time. The symptoms must be persistent and of at least a half year's duration; and have a functional impact on the child or those around him. Unlike many other disorders, the symptoms of ODD do not need to manifest in multiple settings—needing to occur only with at least one other person than a sibling. Forty-three percent of children diagnosed with ODD go on to later meet criteria for conduct disorder (McVoy and Findling 2013).

- *Conduct disorder (CD).* Children with CD are more frequently overtly hostile and law breaking. These people violate the rights of others, such as with bullying or intimidating others, starting fights, using a weapon capable of serious harm such as a brick, fire setting with intent to cause damage, mugging, physical cruelty to others or animals, or stealing, etc. An additional "specifier" exists for the minority of such persons who also demonstrates a lack of remorse, a callous lack of empathy, a lack of concern about their own performance, or shallow affect. In contrast to ODD, people with CD do not show emotional dysregulation. Conduct disorder is associated with a wide range of co-morbidities, including learning disabilities (LDs) and communication disorders. In adulthood, 70–90% go on to meet criteria for antisocial personality disorder (McVoy and Findling 2013).

- *Antisocial personality disorder.* As the person with conduct disorder approaches 18 years of age, he may meet criteria for antisocial personality disorder. People with this disorder have a pervasive pattern of severe violation of the rights of others, typically severe enough to merit arrest. They may be deceitful, impulsive, aggressive, reckless (without regard to safety of others or self), irresponsible at work or to financial obligations, and/or lacking in remorse.

Fortunately the vast majority of the disruptive behavioral disorders fall into the ODD group. The others—conduct disorder and antisocial personality disorder—are beyond the scope of this book.

ODD *through the lifetime*

About 2–16% of people meet criteria for ODD. By puberty, the prevalence of ODD in girls catches up to the prevalence in boys (Lubit 2013).

As infants and toddlers, the ODD child may display irritability, stubbornness, rigidity, aggression, intense reactions, and tantrums. Sometimes, these behaviors are worsened by inconsistent or excessively harsh parenting techniques, or by family stresses. Behavioral symptoms may be so dominant that other underlying problems (such as LD) may be overlooked.

By school age, symptoms may spill over to impact teachers, other adults, and peers. Argumentativeness and poor social skills lead to increasing rejection and attention-seeking behaviors. The children often misinterpret peer actions. Since ODD children often do not see their own role in the problem, they frequently blame others instead. This failure to take responsibility for their actions is a further source of bewilderment and anger for those around them. As the child ages, the earlier symptoms of open defiance may be accompanied by covert activities such as stealing or lying.

Even with maximum intervention, this symptom complex may be difficult to correct—an aggressive toddler is more likely to be an aggressive adult. Those children with particularly intense symptoms as toddlers, and for whom behaviors worsen through early childhood, are at greater risk of developing the more severe conduct disorder in later years. Parental strife, exposure to abuse, and substance abuse can exacerbate the problems.

Relationship with other disorders

ODD is really a symptom complex that potentially can be diagnosed by itself, but more typically occurs in the setting of other diagnoses, such as attention deficit hyperactivity disorder (ADHD), bipolar disorder (BD), depression, or anxiety.

ODD and ADHD

In fact, 50% of ADHD children are said to have Oppositional Defiant Disorder (Lubit 2013). Even in the absence of a full diagnosis, the lives of many children with ADHD are afflicted by lying, cursing, taking things that do not belong to them, blaming others, and being easily angered or annoyed.

This frequency is not surprising given the executive dysfunction seen in so many ADHD children. ADHD people have trouble inhibiting their behavior, anticipating consequences, and learning from their mistakes. No wonder, then, that they keep bumping unpleasantly into other people. Typically, though, we get the sense that these problems are happening "to" the ADHD child. Also, the negative behaviors tend to be more impulsive in ADHD than with ODD. For example, an ADHD child may curse when called for a delicious dinner that his parent has made for him. Most likely, that stems from being overwhelmed with the frustration of making a transition. In ODD, the negative behaviors often seem "deliberately" designed just to achieve the thrill of being negative or difficult. An ODD child would curse when called for dinner more likely because he really intends to worsen the life of his parents— to the degree that a child can be blamed for "intending" anything.

In addition, children with ADHD are usually remorseful (at least, later) compared with ODD kids.

Most children—including those with ADHD—instinctively choose to please others when they can. When the negative behaviors, such as lying, come simply from being overwhelmed, or from the inability to get past the current frustration, I tend to classify them as part of the expanded spectrum of ADHD symptoms. Defined this way, I personally classify relatively few children with ODD.

ODD and depression, anxiety, obsessive-compulsive disorder (OCD), and BD

Depressed and anxious children may suffer from episodes of very threatening low self-esteem. When demands are placed upon them, they may feel "backed into a corner." Their overwhelmed nervous system responds with the "fight or flight" reaction. For children with autistic spectrum disorders (ASDs), anxiety is often such a trigger of oppositional behaviors. Once again, we see that conditions in the syndrome mix can mimic, cause, and exacerbate each other.

Treatment

There are some common-sense interventions that parents and teachers can use to ameliorate the symptoms of ODD.

☐ *Evaluate and treat any underlying or associated problems*, such as ADHD, BD, depression, OCD/anxiety, ASD, or LD that can underlie or worsen the problem. *This is critical.*

☐ *See the suggestions in Chapter 2*—in particular, Rule 2.

» Pick your battles.

» Head off fights before they happen.

» Stay calm!

» Do not engage in "discussion" with an out-of-control brain (yours or the child's). Wait until tempers have abated.

☐ *Don't show negative emotions* to the child's behavior. That just reinforces it. Either ignore the child's negative comments, or calmly hand out the previously established punishment for the infraction.

☐ *Decide how you will respond to problems before they occur.* The planned response is much more likely to be reasonable and helpful than a response made in the heat of the moment (see Jim Chandler's website in Further Reading section).

☐ *Choose reasonable punishments* that actually teach a lesson, and that can actually be enforced.

☐ *Find something positive* to praise and focus on. Reward flexibility and cooperation.

It is also important to take care of yourself (with good sleep, eating, and fun times for yourself) and to take care of your relationships with others, as the ODD child will exploit any weaknesses in those relationships. The psychiatrist Dr. Jim Chandler (see Further Reading section), amongst his other excellent suggestions, implores that we *do not believe what the child with ODD says about others*. ODD kids are masters at assigning blame onto other people. Parents are told incorrect, horrible stories about teachers; fathers about mothers; and vice versa. Everyone involved in an ODD child's life needs to talk *directly* with each other!

☐ *Discuss the need for direct communication in advance of any problems.*

☐ *Schedule regular meetings* between the school and parents.

☐ *Confirm everything with direct communication.*

Another good idea is to limit "screen time." Screen time refers to any activity that has a screen, such as TV, videogames, computer games, texting, and the internet. These activities can be clearly addicting, often teach negative behaviors, may agitate the kids, and it is difficult to get kids to stop using them. The American Academy of Pediatrics (2014) recommends limiting non-educational media time to two hours per day. It is true, though, that holding screen time as a reward for good behavior can be a powerful tool.

If symptoms are worsening rather than improving, professional help should be sought. Problems are most responsive when interventions begin at an earlier age. Options include:

☐ *professional help* for the treatment of co-occurring ADHD, depression, LD, etc.

☐ *family counseling* (to improve communication and examine the issue of exposure to violence or abuse)

☐ *parental management training* (to help break the downhill spiral of parent/child interactions)

☐ *social skills group training* (to learn flexibility and improve the child's tolerance of peers)

☐ *cognitive behavioral therapy* (to learn problem-solving skills)

☐ *individual psychotherapy.*

There is evidence that parental management training for the parents, along with social skills group training for the children, work well together. However, relatively little research has been done on the most effective management techniques. Apparently, researchers avoid ODD children just like other people may do.

Medication

There are no medications that directly change your "attitude." However, medications are often needed to treat the underlying or co-occurring parts of the syndrome mix that are triggering the ODD symptoms. Medication may be used to great effect in the treatment of ADHD, depression, BD, or anxiety disorders.

Medications such as alpha-2 agonists (e.g., Tenex and Catapres); mood stabilizers (e.g., Depakote, Lamictal, and Tegretol); and atypical neuroleptics (such as Risperdal) can sometimes help with impulsivity and aggression. These are discussed in Chapter 14.

Intermittent explosive disorder

This DSM-5 disorder (APA 2013) is marked by aggressive outbursts that are:

- based on an inability to control impulsive or angry *reactions* (i.e., are not premeditated nor have an ulterior motive such as being designed to intimidate)

- out of proportion to the precipitating trigger

- demonstrating verbal aggression (tantrums, verbal fights) or mild physical aggression (not resulting in actual damage or harm) occurring an average of two times/week

- additionally demonstrating more severe outbursts (causing physical damage or harm) occurring at least three times/year.

The child must be at least six years of age, and the outbursts must result in significant problems with functioning. They typically last fewer than 30 minutes.

Treatment recommendations tend to follow those for oppositional defiant disorder.

Sorting out conditions that have behavioral explosions

As we have seen, there are a number of conditions of the syndrome mix that are either primarily defined by, or perhaps associated with, explosive behaviors and/or mood problems. These conditions are each discussed in their own chapter, but are compared with each other below (APA 2013, p.468).

- Behavioral explosions as defining features:

  ◦ *intermittent explosive disorder* is defined by impulsive (not spiteful) outbursts with relatively *normal mood in between*. They can be physical or verbal, and have a wide range of triggers

- *disruptive mood dysregulation disorder* is defined by impulsive outbursts with *persistently negative mood in between* outbursts.

• Behavioral explosions as part of other conditions:

- *ADHD* (outbursts are impulsive and directed at whoever is in the room)

- *oppositional defiant disorder* (outbursts are directed at authority figures, are frequently spiteful, and are not physical—in distinction to intermittent explosive disorders, which have a wide range of triggers, are not spiteful, and can be both verbal and physical)

- *conduct disorder* (outbursts are proactive and predatory)

- *major depressive episode* (outbursts occur during discrete episodes of depression)

- *bipolar disorders* (outbursts occur during the discrete episodes of mania, hypomania and/or depression).

See also Table 10.1 on page 210.

CHAPTER 13

Central Auditory Processing Disorders (CAPDs)

Teacher: "Okay, class. Be quiet, go to your seats, take out your math book, open to page 46, and do every other problem starting with question number 3."

Pause. John gets lost after, "Be quiet."

Teacher: "John, you haven't even opened your book yet—even though I know you are good at math. Didn't you get what I just said? Don't you care?"

What happened?

What is central auditory processing?

When a sound vibration hits our eardrum, a series of small bones in our middle ear transmits the information to nerve receptors located in our inner ear. These receptors send the raw information towards our brain via the auditory nerves. Central auditory processing (CAP), like its name says, is the central nervous system's processing (of that unrefined auditory information coming from our auditory nerves) into something useful. In its simplest terms, CAP is the analysis and interpretation of information from our ears or, "what we do with what the ear hears."

Central auditory processing disorders (CAPDs), then, are problems with one or more aspects of the CAP process. CAPD is not a single disease entity, but rather a group of problems that can occur singly or in combination. This group of conditions is sometimes also called APDs—auditory processing disorders. CAPD is felt to occur in about 2–3% of the population, with boys outnumbering girls by 2:1 (Schminky and Baran 1999).

So much for the simple answers. Now, let's examine in some more detail the specific processes involved in processing noise once you have detected it. Note that these steps overlap and are inseparable. Do not be thrown off by the fancy terms—they mean just what they say.

- *Discrimination*—the ability to discriminate the different pitch, duration, and intensity (loudness) of the sounds. This essential hearing task will affect progress in virtually all academic skills.

- *Auditory discrimination*—the ability to discriminate (distinguish) between words that sound similar to each other, such as between "hip" and "hit." Importantly, background noise makes this process significantly harder for children with CAPD.

- *Localization*—the ability to determine where a sound is coming from; and, thus, where you should direct your attention.

- *Auditory attention*—the ability to sustain attention to that sound.

- *Auditory figure-ground*—the ability to separate out the primary sound (the "figure," such as the teacher's voice) from the background sound (the "ground," such as other noise in the classroom). Imagine your own experience listening to a friend at a noisy party. Imagine if your whole day was like that.

- *Auditory closure*—the process whereby we can still understand the whole word or message even if part of it is missing or degraded. Our nervous system has a great deal of redundancy built in, and can usually fill in the gaps (i.e., provide "closure"). Again, consider your experience at a noisy party. You can carry on a complete conversation without even hearing much of what the other person is saying.

- *Auditory synthesis*—the ability to synthesize/blend isolated phonemes (sounds) into words. An example would be blending the sounds "puh"—"uh"—"te" together to form the word pronounced "put." Clearly, this is an essential step in reading.

- *Auditory analysis*—the ability to identify parts of words embedded within the word (for example, help*s* versus help*ed*). In particular, this skill is essential to develop verb tenses.

- *Auditory association*—the ability to attach a meaning, once we have isolated and refined the noise into a word or specific sound. Frankly, it is astounding that most of us have the instant ability to know that the sound "h—o—t" means "something that could burn you."

- *Auditory memory*—the ability to store and later recall what we have heard.

Other needed skills, but that are not unique to auditory processing, include attention, language, and memory.

All of these CAP steps happen on the sensory (input) side of language—occurring particularly in our brainstem and temporal lobes. This must all occur before we can even get to the other cognitive processes accomplished by the rest of the brain: figuring out the answer to what we just heard, expressing the answer, and acting upon our answer. It is amazing that any of us can communicate at all.

Diagnosing CAPD

Symptoms

Given all of the component skills that are encompassed by the initials CAPD, it is not surprising that there is a large shopping list of possible symptoms. The following list includes some of the warning signs to make us *consider* the diagnosis of CAPD, and possibly undertake further testing. Making matters worse, once again, is the high frequency in which CAPD co-occurs, mimics, and worsens other conditions of the syndrome mix covered in this book, such as attention deficit hyperactivity disorder (ADHD) and language problems.

Consider CAPD when a student shows:

- difficulty with hearing in a noisy environment, or over the phone

- difficulty when competing noises scramble comprehension (all of us have to work harder to *hear* the main speaker when the room gets noisy, but CAPD kids may have to work harder to *understand* in a noisy room; it is as if the competing noise not only drowns out the teacher's voice, but also turns on an eggbeater and scrambles it)

- unusual sensitivity or complaints about noise

- difficulty telling the direction from which someone is talking

- difficulty sustaining and directing attention, especially against competing noises

- difficulty following multi-step directions, especially if given in one sentence

- difficulty following long conversations

- difficulty remembering information presented aurally (people with CAPD may prefer viewing videos with the written subtitles turned on)

- confusion over words with similar sounds

- difficulty learning a foreign language or uncommon vocabulary words

- lack of awareness of the speaker

- lack of understanding ("I heard you, but I don't know what you mean")

- difficulty with organization

- non-verbal problems (such as music appreciation)

- verbal IQ (intelligence quotient) lower than performance IQ

- poor performance in auditory-based psycho-educational tests

- reading, spelling, or speech problems (if the child does not hear words properly, then all tasks based initially on phonics are at risk)

- unexplained poor academic performance

- hearing loss.

Distinguishing CAPD from ADHD

It is easy to confuse CAPD and ADHD (especially of the inattentive type) as they can co-occur with each other and share:

- difficulty paying attention

- difficulty telling the foreground from the background noise

- difficulty with following a sequence of directions.

We can note some distinguishing features, though, in Table 13.1.

TABLE 13.1: Distinguishing features of ADHD and CAPD

ADHD	CAPD
Difficulty attending to all non-intriguing tasks.	Difficulty attending to listening-related tasks
Background noise makes it harder to attend to the information.	Background noise scrambles the information.
Students typically can understand, once you get their attention.	Students may have trouble with comprehension of oral tasks, even once you get their attention.
Executive function difficulties.	Executive function relatively intact, as long as the child understands the task at hand.
May be physically hyperactive, over-reactive, or impulsive.	Unless acting out from academic frustration, students are not usually disruptive.
Typically do not have memory problems.	May have auditory memory problems.

Testing

As we can see, the warning symptoms for potential CAPD are quite variable, and some are not very specific. Once the diagnosis is considered, we need further testing—even though that is still not perfect. Full CAPD testing requires specialized equipment, and is typically done by an audiologist or speech therapist with particular training in the area.

Typically, children need to be seven years old before the testing is reliable, although some tests can be done by age five. In addition, results are difficult to interpret in children with low IQ, language problems, or ADHD. CAPD testing is usually done as part of a larger psycho-educational evaluation. The child's clinical symptoms help to guide the choice of tests.

The following descriptions will help you to understand these specialized tests, and to better understand the particular problems that they test for.

- *Baseline audiometric peripheral hearing test—"a hearing test."* The first step is to be sure that the child is actually capable of hearing sounds at different frequencies and volumes. A hearing loss does not preclude the possibility of a CAPD, but certainly makes testing for it more difficult.

- *Brainstem auditory evoked responses (BAER)*. This test is like a mini-EEG (electroencephalogram). Sounds are played into earphones, which evoke responses from the child's nervous system. Electrodes are placed on the child's head to check for any delay of these electrical impulses as they work their way through the brainstem and the rest of the brain.

- *Monaural low redundancy speech tests.* In these tests, the sounds are presented "monaurally," i.e., to one ear at a time. The sounds are degraded—by cutting out part of the sounds electronically, changing their frequency, etc. This lowers the normal redundancy that we depend upon to figure out the word. These tests stress the system, and check how well the student can figure out and complete sounds ("auditory closure").

- *Dichotic speech tests.* Here, different sounds are presented to each ear, either simultaneously or in an overlapping manner. The child repeats the words. He may be asked to say everything he heard, which tests his listening even when his attention is divided amongst multiple sources ("divided attention"). Or he may have to say only what he heard from one ear, which tests how well he can direct his attention ("directed attention"). Try out a dichotic test at www.linguistics.ucla.edu/people/schuh/lx001/Dichotic/dichotic.html (but don't let your child who is going to be tested try it—it may have a "practice effect" on the official test).

- *Temporal patterning tests.* The ability to process the pattern of non-verbal sounds is checked in this group of tests. For example, the child may be asked to hum a pattern of sounds that she heard, or to describe the pattern.

- *Binaural integration/interaction tests.* Different parts of the speech signal are presented to different ears, and the child's ability to integrate those signals into a single sound is tested. For example, a "d" sound is played into the right ear while an "og" sound is played into the left ear. A typical child would have no difficulty blending these sounds into "dog."

Treatments at home and school

There is no single set of recommendations that applies to this diverse group of difficulties. A specific plan needs to be made for the set of deficits diagnosed in each child. Treatments include modifying the environment, working directly on the deficit, and circumventing the deficit. Many of the following suggestions come from an excellent Technical Assistance Paper from the Florida Department of Education (2001).

Ensure appropriate seating

☐ **Seat the child near the action.** Preferably, place the student three to four feet from the main action, but up to six to eight feet away is okay. This will allow the child to maximize visual and audio cues, as well as help with attention. As the focus of the class moves, the child may need to move as well. However, we also need to do the following things:

  » Avoid competing noises! As we have seen, background noises can scramble the signal for CAPD children. Avoid doorways, noisy window areas, bubbling fish tanks, humming lights, nearby bathrooms, etc.

  » Provide a quiet, private study area if needed—both in school and at home.

  » Provide mufflers/ear plugs if needed. In order to minimize any stigma, allow other children to use mufflers as well.

Get and keep the child's attention

☐ *Get the child's visual and auditory attention.* This will allow for maximal use of multisensory learning, which is essential for students who have problems with information coming through one sense.

☐ *Establish eye contact when speaking* (unless this is uncomfortable for the child). At home, turn off the television; and be sure that you are in the same room as the child while you are talking.

☐ *Cue the children with directives* such as "THIS IS IMPORTANT!" or "Remember this!"

☐ *Mark transition periods clearly* with appropriate advance warnings and directions for the new task.

☐ *Use predictable daily routines.*

☐ *Provide help with note taking.* It may be difficult to pay attention to the teacher, the teacher's voice, and take notes all at the same time.

☐ *Attention issues may be worse at school* due to the commotion. However, they may be worse at home because who can maintain so much effort all day long? Don't blame the child if he listens better at school or at home.

When talking to the child

☐ *Speak clearly, slowly,* and with comfortable loudness.

☐ *Vary your tone of voice and rate of speech* to keep attention and emphasize important material.

☐ *Use natural gestures* that support your words, but are not so excessive that they distract the child.

☐ *Give direct and uncomplicated directions.*

☐ *Give directions one at a time, in order.*

☐ *Allow time to process each direction.*

☐ *Repeat directions as needed,* preferably using simpler language.

☐ *Model/demonstrate the directions* if possible. Teachers can write directions as they say them. Write a list of the steps.

☐ *Don't assume that the child understands the subtle parts of your comments.*

☐ *Encourage the student to ask for clarification,* if needed. Never say, "What, weren't you listening?"

☐ *Check the child's comprehension* by asking her to repeat what she heard using different words.

☐ *Check that the child understands* by monitoring her progress frequently—making sure that the work is being done as directed. This will help avoid the deflating experience of doing a great job at the wrong task.

☐ *Look for "avoidance,"* which may really be a lack of comprehension.

☐ *A low teacher–student ratio* may be helpful.

☐ *A student peer* may help explain material.

Teachers, parents, and the child can all share with each other their insights into how the child learns best.

Use the tactics of preview and review

☐ *Review old material before presenting something new.*

☐ *Preview new material before the primary presentation.* This can be via a brief summary of the new material, or by providing material to review at home before coming to class.

☐ *Show how the information relates to the child's life.*

☐ *Write an outline on the board,* along with new vocabulary.

☐ *Frequently summarize key points,* and ask students for summaries.

☐ *CAPD students may benefit from individualized help.*

Facilitate time management

☐ *Allow extra time*—for tests and for individual classroom responses.

☐ *Break up academic activity* to avoid fatigue.

☐ *Schedule the most intense academic activities in the morning,* for most students.

☐ *Encourage the use of an assignment book and organizer.* Monitor its use!

Teach compensatory techniques

☐ *Encourage the child to use multisensory learning*—such as saying, writing, and visualizing the material to be learned. Some children benefit from pretending to write the material in the air.

☐ *Allow the child to subvocalize,* if needed.

☐ *Teach how to use mnemonics.* For example, we learned how to read music notes on the staff by the mnemonic "F—A—C—E."

☐ *Teach how to use "visual grids"* as hooks from which to hang information. For example, on the left side of the grid are the points in favor of the Democrats, and on the right side are the points in favor of the Republicans. If a child simply remembers which side of the page he saw the fact on, he can assign it to the correct political party. These grids can be written on paper, and later recalled visually to help sort out the information.

☐ *Teach how to chunk information into small sections,* to facilitate memory. For example, rather than remembering six random American history events, divide them into those occurring before the American Revolution and those after. Rather than remembering 243564875, remember 243 564 875.

☐ *Teach how to use spellcheck.*

☐ *Some children might benefit from material being recorded,* but, honestly, who has time to listen to the whole day again?

Classroom adaptations can often help

☐ *FM (frequency modulated) amplifiers may be suggested by the audiologist.* They are useful for those subtypes of CAPD marked by inability to separate the foreground from the background noise, difficulty integrating material, or difficulty organizing information. The system is basically a closed-circuit radio set up. The teacher wears a microphone, and the student wears an earphone, or much better, a speaker magnifies the teacher's voice for the entire class, making it easier to distinguish her voice from background noise. Many students will not tolerate the "stigma" attached to a personal earphone, making the whole room speaker a better choice.

☐ *Improve classroom acoustics with drapes,* carpet, and sound-absorbing wall hangings and bulletin boards. Tennis balls placed under chair legs will reduce noise.

☐ *Arrange the classroom to allow individual and small group settings.*

☐ *Avoid open classrooms.*

There are also many computer programs designed to help CAPD. Recommendation for these may be given as part of the audiologist's report.

CHAPTER 14

Medications

Medicating kids? What is this world coming to?

Before we can discuss the individual medications, we need to address a more basic question: Is it ethical to give psychoactive medications to children?

Let's begin with a brief survey, to clarify what group of children we are discussing. Raise your hand if you are in favor of the following:

- A child who has no problem gets no medicine. (I assume we are all raising our hands. Certainly, I am.)

- A child who has a problem that can be handled without medication gets no medication. (Again, I assume we are all raising our hands.) Now, for the big question.

- A child who has a neurologically based problem, and behavioral interventions have been unable to preserve his happiness, gets medication to see if it can help. (I hope that, given these qualifications, we are raising our hands as well.)

When a child is brought to my medical office, it is almost never the first step. Enticements, bribes, threats, pretending that it will soon go away, and prayer have been tried first. It is great if those interventions are successful. However, if they have not succeeded in preserving the child's self-esteem, then I invoke the following basic strategy: "If it's working, keep doing it. If it's not, do something else." Sometimes, that something else is medication.

Benefits of medication

In the bad old days, there was little distinction between epilepsy, migraines (with their weird vision attacks followed by dropping to the floor in pain), witchcraft, and psychiatric disease. Mercifully, the Dark Age concepts of epilepsy and migraines have been largely dropped in modern times. Most of us do not think of people with epilepsy as being possessed, or weak of spirit. It's brain biochemistry. We don't tell them to, "Just get your act together and stop seizuring!" It currently makes perfect sense to use anticonvulsants for seizures, just like it makes sense to use insulin for diabetes when diet does not work.

Unfortunately, many of us are still a few centuries behind when it comes to psychiatric disease. MRI (magnetic resonance imaging) scans, PET (positron emission tomography) scans, adoption studies, and more, show the biochemical basis of much of psychiatric disease. When behavioral and environmental interventions do not work, it makes sense to use biochemical interventions, i.e., medications, for biochemical problems.

People with attention deficit hyperactivity disorder (ADHD), obsessive-compulsive disorder (OCD), bipolar disorder (BD), Tourette's syndrome, etc. did not ask to have their problems. It has nothing to do with lack of will power.

What if they discover something bad about these drugs?

No one can guarantee that, 50 years from now, there might not be some side effect that we do not know about currently. Many of these medications already do have a long record of apparent safety, such as stimulants that have been used for about half a century (although few long-term controlled follow-up studies have been done). Other medications have quite limited experience in children. When possible, we use the safest medication with the longest safety record. We try to navigate the best course. There are no guarantees in life. Life has risks.

For some children, though, there is a risk associated with *not* using medication. There are often huge difficulties for these children if we cannot help them get on the right track—problems with poor school performance, unhappiness, and substance abuse. By the time these children are being considered for medication, they are often well on the road to these risks—and getting deeper into these problems.

So when we talk about the possible risks of medication, it needs to be weighed against the risks of no medication. For some children, the known immediate risk of their condition outweighs a possible unknown medical one.

Don't these drugs lead to substance abuse?

Many people fear that the use of psychoactive drugs in children will lead to future substance abuse. Actually, most all of the evidence points to the opposite. Multiple studies have shown that stimulant treatment for ADHD cuts the risk of future substance abuse by more than half (e.g., Wilens *et al.* 2003), although a recent editorial (Goldstein 2013, p.226) states that the best that can be currently stated with confidence is that, "stimulants *may* decrease the risk of substance misuse for some youth with ADHD." In other words, there *may* be a large *protective effect* of stimulants against substance abuse. Research has not shown yet *why* stimulants may lower the risk of substance abuse in ADHD people; but presumably, those people who are now able to find success in society have less need to seek alternate forms of pleasure or escape. It is actually fair to ask, "How can we withhold a treatment, when withholding the treatment may double the child's risk for substance abuse?" This is not to say, though, that stimulants and other medications can't be abused.

How will people ever learn to handle their own problems if they rely on medication?

Once again, medications are to be added after attempts to get the child to "handle" his own problem have already failed, or to make those interventions more likely to succeed. The medications may be needed to give the child the basic tools that he needs to comply with behavioral approaches. For example, once you have given a child a reasonable attention span, then we can ask him to behave in class.

"But aren't we being too soft on these kids?" No! They are already having a tough life, and even on medication, their life will still be tougher than is typical. By the time medication is prescribed, the person will have already been struggling with these issues far more than typical people. The medications are not perfect. The difficulty will continue, but it will now be a tolerable and fair fight. There will still be plenty of opportunity to build character.

Attitudes to medications

Let's not confuse being "famous" with being "infamous." Drugs such as Ritalin and Prozac have garnered a lot of press. Many people think that "famous" must mean "bad." We should remember, though, that drugs usually only make it to the front cover of a magazine because they are used frequently. In turn, they are only used frequently because they are effective and relatively safe. Just because you have heard about a medication, it does not mean that it is a bad medication.

Who makes the decision to use medications?

Ultimately, the choice to use medication is made by the family, the child, and the physician. We depend—often quite significantly—upon data from a multitude of sources, including the school. Teachers and other school professionals are our eyes and ears. However, medical decisions are made between the child's family and doctor.

Doctors also depend upon the frontline observers (parents and teachers) to let us know if and when the medication is working, and if and when side effects are seen.

International differences

Clearly, different medications are used with different frequency in different countries. This probably has more to do with different diagnostic criteria, societal views on medication, and societal expectations than with actual differences in rates of the disorders. The brand names and the indications for drug usage contained in this book are given from a US common practice perspective. Behavioral, other non-pharmacological, and homeopathic treatments are discussed in each of the preceding chapters.

> This information—as is the information in the rest of this book—is not intended to be all-inclusive, and does not constitute medical advice, which can only be obtained on an individualized basis by a properly licensed physician or other professional. Note that the pediatric and/or adult use of some of these medications has not been formally approved by the US Food and Drug Administration (FDA) for either a given age range of patient or a particular indication. Information and recommendations regarding use and monitoring of medications are subject to debate and future changes. Follow updates with your professionals and at www.fda.gov. Always check with your pharmacist or doctor before taking these or any other medications, especially checking for any drug interactions. Always read information given out by your pharmacist.

Further information can be found at the resources listed in the Further Reading section. In particular, see the following websites:

- www.drugs.com covers all medications with information for the general public and also at the professional level. See also their drug interaction checker and pill identifier resources.

- www.parentsmedguide.org contains fantastic guides focused on the medication treatments of ADHD, depression, and bipolar. Prepared by the American Psychiatric Association and the American Academy of Child and Adolescent Psychiatry.

Medications for ADHD

Stimulants: an overview

The medications commonly referred to as "stimulants" have the longest and best track record in treating ADHD. They increase levels of the brain transmitters dopamine and norepinephrine. This wakes up the frontal lobes, so that they can now do a better job at executive functions such as inhibiting distractions and impulsivity.

As we saw in Chapter 3, ADHDers are like bicycles without brakes. They careen around, unable to go anywhere but where gravity takes them. The stimulants are analogous to waking up the bicycle's brake linings. Stimulants are *not* like sedatives. Sedatives would be analogous to pouring tar on the bike's gears—making the child too tired to bother anyone. That would be a horrible thing to do. Stimulants, again, are just the opposite. They make a higher-performing bike—one with self-control. The kids still have the same sparkle in their eye, they're just able to sit and do one thing at a time. The occasional child who get a "flattening" effect (which I call a "loss of bubbles") can usually be handled by lowering the dose or switching medication.

There is nothing paradoxical about stimulants having a "calming" effect in children or adults. In a person of any age, they function the same: the person sits still because she is now properly awake, not because she is sedated. It works in the same fashion as adults who take coffee. Secretaries "quiet down" after coffee break and start typing because they are now awake and alert, not because they are too tired from the coffee to chat anymore.

Observant students notice that they get their work done more efficiently, and, for some reason, people seem to yell at them less. However, they don't feel anything, any more than people "feel" anything when they wear their glasses. Patients seem to notice when they are not on it, more than feel "different" on it. After all, normalcy has no feeling. Some of my favorite patient comments about how they felt on stimulants are listed here.

- "My brain gets plugged in. My silly brain gets pushed away by my smart brain."

- "I feel sorry for the kids who now get into the trouble that I used to."

- "At 7pm, my Adderall packs its bags and says 'Goodbye!' for the night."

- "I don't know how it makes me feel. I wasn't paying attention!"

Objective studies show that other people do notice a significant difference. A recent meta-analysis (a study combining the results of multiple other studies) showed that students increased their on-task behavior and the amount of schoolwork that they were able to complete by factors of up to 15% (Prasad 2013). Improvements in actual grades have been less consistently demonstrated, but the medications may be most helpful in math (Prasad 2013).

Another area where stimulant medications seem to help is driving. People with ADHD are at a significantly higher risk of driving accidents. Fortunately, a recent simulator study showed that ADHD patients treated with Vyvanse (lisdexamfetamine) for five weeks were 67% less likely to have a collision during a driving simulation than those who received a placebo (Beiderman 2012). As they say, "Don't leave home without it." While we're on the subject of car safety, stress the dangers of distracted driving such as texting. Texting is a double whammy for people with ADHD. A pledge not to text while driving, along with links to helpful cell phone apps, can be found at www.itcanwait.com.

Methylphenidate preparations (short-acting)

- *Ritalin* contains the "gold standard" of stimulants—methylphenidate, which is the generic name of the active chemical in Ritalin. Ritalin tablets last only about two to five hours. Thus, Ritalin requires frequent dosing, including the infamous trip to the school nurse at lunchtime. Even the lunch dose of Ritalin wears out by homework time, leading to frequent fights with parents over homework. Rebound—a transient period of nasty, irrational, and tearful behavior occurring as the medication level drops rapidly at the end of its time span—has been most common with the short-acting preparations.

- *Focalin (dexmethylphenidate)* is just the active part of methylphenidate (just the d-isomer). It seems to last a little longer than regular Ritalin, and requires only half of the dose.

Methylphenidate preparations (long-acting)

Long-lasting preparations of methylphenidate are replacing traditional short-acting forms. Although swallowed once in the morning, these formulations keep releasing the medication throughout the day. This saves children from going to the nurse at lunchtime, and some preparations last long enough to allow more children to benefit from medication effect during homework time—a practice that is clearly recommended. These preparations also seem to have less rebound. In addition, when compared with the easily crushable short-acting tablets, abuse of the long-acting preparations is less likely, since the paste or beads they employ are harder to abuse.

- *Concerta.* This was the first good, long-acting preparation of methylphenidate to be marketed. It approximates the release of three doses of methylphenidate, giving it an effective life of about ten+ hours. The first dose is contained in the outer coating of the capsule, and is released within the first hour. Inside the capsule is a sponge, which absorbs fluid from the gastrointestinal tract. The expanding sponge then slowly pushes two separate doses of medication out of the other end of the capsule. Concerta is designed to release 22% of the total daily dose in the morning, and the higher 78% proportion of medication later in the day.

- *Daytrana Patch.* This preparation releases methylphenidate into the bloodstream by way of a patch adhered to the skin each morning. An advantage is that it can be removed at any point up to nine hours (and will continue to work several more hours after being removed). This gives the family more control over the medication's duration of action. However, it takes several minutes to apply, can be removed by the child, and can cause skin irritation or possibly even allergy to the adhesive or even the medication itself. Given all of the other options that also do not involve swallowing an intact pill, Daytrana is not a usual first-line choice.

- *Focalin XR.* This capsule contains beads that split the total dose of Focalin into two parts, 50% delivered early and the other 50% delivered four hours later. The capsules can be swallowed whole or sprinkled on a spoonful of applesauce.

- *Metadate CD.* This capsule uses beads that release their methylphenidate at different times, to approximate a twice a day dosage. Metadate CD is designed to release about 30% of its medication early and the remaining 70% later during the day. The capsules can be opened and sprinkled on applesauce.

- *Ritalin LA.* This capsule is an effective preparation that should not be confused with the older Ritalin SR, which is the previous, less effective wax matrix release formulation. The Ritalin LA capsules can be opened and sprinkled on applesauce. The capsules release 50% of the medication quickly, and the other 50% about four hours later.

- *Quillivant* is a fairly new liquid preparation of methylphenidate, with the unique quality of being *a long-acting liquid* medication. Great care must be given to shaking the bottle carefully before each use, as the active ingredient might not otherwise be evenly distributed in the liquid.

Dextro-amphetamine preparations

- *Dexedrine tablets* (with a four-hour effect) and *Dexedrine spansules* (with a ten-hour effect) are the brand names for dextro-amphetamine preparations.

- *Vyvanse (lisdexamfetamine)* is a variant of dextro-amphetamine, where the amino acid lysine (which we eat all day as a building block of proteins) is attached to the dextro-amphetamine molecule. This entire structure only becomes neurologically active when the person's own metabolism splits off the amino acid, thereby freeing the active amphetamine molecule. So, even if the person abuses the powder by snorting it, etc. right into the blood-stream, the medication will still only have a gradual onset and course of action as the body slowly metabolizes it into its active form. It has thus been presented as a good choice in populations prone to substance abuse or diversion. It also seems to work a little longer than the other long-acting preparations. The Vyvanse capsule may be swallowed intact, or the contents may be dissolved into a small glass of water.

Mixed amphetamine salt preparations

- *Adderall tablets* (with a four to six-hour effect) and *Adderall XR spansules* (with a ten+ hour effect) have become common choices in the treatment of ADHD—especially the XR form. Adderall is a mixture of different kinds of dextro- and levo-amphetamine. The capsules can be opened and sprinkled on applesauce or swallowed intact.

Which stimulant to use?

As of this writing, there is no consensus as to the best stimulant preparation, although some doctors feel that methylphenidate compounds are slightly more "gentle," and amphetamine compounds are slightly more effective. Most experts would agree, though, that:

- the long-lasting preparations are preferable to the short-acting ones

- if one class of stimulants does not work, or causes side effects, then trial with another preparation should be considered

- if a long-lasting preparation still does not last long enough, then a short-acting preparation can be added at the end of the afternoon

- most children benefit from the use of medication during homework time; and if medication allows the child to get better feedback on weekends/vacations, then it can be used at those times as well.

Possible side effects of stimulants

Considering how effective they can be, the stimulants are usually quite well tolerated. Most children "feel nothing" when they take it. However, there are possible side effects.

- Loss of appetite (particularly for lunch) is a common issue, but occurs in only a fraction of kids.

- Insomnia is the other common issue, but again occurs in only a fraction of children. See Appendix 3 for sleep hygiene treatment recommendations for insomnia.

- Headache.

- Rebound occurs in some children as the medication level drops too rapidly at the end of the pill's duration, i.e., typically around 3pm to 5pm. Rebound is a pretty characteristic syndrome where the child becomes uncharacteristically irritable, irrational, and tearful—not just a return to his pre-medication self. For example, there may be a big fight about Mom having bought the wrong kind of pencil. Half an hour later, it's all over, leaving everyone bewildered. We can tell that it's not a direct effect of the working medication because that would happen in mid-morning, when the medication level is peaking. Check to make sure that the "rebound" is not actually due to hunger secondary to poor appetite at lunch. Rebound can be handled by: staying out of each other's way until the irritability passes; by a tiny touch-up dose of a short-acting preparation given shortly before the rebound usually occurs; or by switching to another preparation (typically long-acting), which may have a more gradual wear down period.

• Tics can be worsened, unchanged, or improved during the time period when stimulants are employed. Contrary to package insert warnings and previous common perception, as a whole, the field is moving towards the view that methylphenidate compounds can be used safely for *most* children with ADHD and tics. In one study (Tourettes Syndrome Study Group 2002), for example, 136 children with ADHD and chronic tics were randomly assigned to different treatments. The percent worsening of the tics was the same whether drugs or placebo was given:

  ◦ methylphenidate treatment: 20% worsened

  ◦ clonidine (typically treats tics): 26% worsened

  ◦ placebo ("sugar pill"): 22% worsened.

Further, the overall group severity of tics actually decreased in all actively treated groups. In particular, though, especially supra-therapeutic doses of amphetamines are preferentially avoided in children with co-morbid ADHD and tics.

• Stimulants do not seem to "stunt your growth." Most children have less than an inch of height difference while they are on the medication. Usually, the rate of height and weight growth returns to normal over time. Research is not clear about whether the stimulants actually affect ultimate height. Any child who is not following her expected growth pattern over time should have consideration of a medical/endocrine evaluation, regardless of whether or not she is on stimulants. After all, being on stimulants does not protect a child from growth hormone deficiency or other cause of failure to grow.

- Stimulants may provoke mania or possibly worsen other behaviors.

- Note that although stimulants have been felt to be contraindicated in ADHD with co-morbid anxiety disorder, recent evidence actually shows that one out of five such children have meaningful reduction in their anxiety when stimulants are used for their ADHD (Tannock 2009, p.143).

- Discuss cardiac warnings and appropriate evaluations for all stimulants with your doctor. Note that children treated long term with stimulants have pulse increases of one to five beats/minute and blood pressure increases of one to five mm of mercury; up to 15% of children will show greater effects than that (Hammerness 2011). Most studies do *not* show an increased risk of serious cardiovascular events such as sudden death when compared with children who are not on stimulants.

- New warnings have been posted regarding possible circulation problems in fingers and toes (peripheral vasculopathy, including Raynaud's phenomenon). Fingers or toes may feel numb, cool, or painful, and may change from pale, to blue, to red. Tell your doctor about any of these symptoms, and call your doctor right away if your child has any unexplained wounds on the fingers or toes.

- The FDA has recently released a warning for the rare risk of priapism (sustained penile erection) with ADHD medications including methylphenidate products and atomoxetine (Strattera). An erection lasting four hours is a medical emergency requiring immediate emergency room intervention.

- Stimulants are extremely unlikely to cause systemic problems such as liver or bone marrow.

- As we have seen above, multiple studies show that stimulants as prescribed do not increase the risk of future substance abuse, and in fact, may lower the risk.

- Possible *misuse* of medication (either incorrect dosage or using stimulants that are not prescribed to the child) occurs in up to 9% of high school and younger children, and up to 35% of college students. Of those 35% of college misusers, half said they took it to study better, and one-third said they took it to get high or experiment (Wilens *et al.* 2008).

- Possible *diversion* of medication (transfer to another person) occurs in 16% of grade and high school students, and 23% of college students; wherein the ADHD youngsters are approached to give, buy, or trade their stimulant meds (Wilens *et al.* 2008). Children should be aware that not only is it incredibly dangerous and stupid, but it is also a US federal offense to even *give* a controlled substance to a friend, or for the friend to possess it without his own prescription. ADHDers with co-morbid conduct disorder and/or substance use disorder are at particularly high risk for selling or misusing their medications (Prince and Wilens 2009, p.364). The FDA clearly warns of the abuse potential of stimulant medications.

Non-stimulants for ADHD

Nothing works for ADHD as well as the stimulants. However, a "non-stimulant" may be suggested by your doctor in the 20% of cases where stimulants are either ineffective, contraindicated, or not tolerated. Non-stimulants have no direct effect on the neurotransmitter dopamine. That's both good and bad: it's "good" because dopamine has its side effects such as addiction potential; it's "bad" because non-stimulants have no direct effect on dopamine (and dopamine is an important player in ADHD).

Non-stimulants appear to have little abuse potential, and may be used preferentially in patients where substance abuse is an issue. Unlike stimulants—which work the first day as well as they ever will at that dose—the non-stimulants may take weeks to months to show their full ADHD effect. The non-stimulants also need to be titrated upwards or downwards slowly, and taken seven days a week—they can't be started and stopped more or less at will as can the stimulants.

- *Strattera* (atomoxetine is the generic name) was released in 2002. Unlike the stimulants, Strattera has direct effect only upon the neurotransmitter norepinephrine. In other words, it has no direct dopaminergic effect. It can cause decreased appetite. Unlike stimulants, Strattera can frequently be sedating when started. Its full effect may not be observed for several weeks or more. Discuss warnings for Strattera regarding possible liver problems, heart problems, very low incidence of thoughts of self-harm (especially when changing doses up or down), and mania with your doctor. Although there are reports of occasional cases of worsening tics occurring at the same time as Strattera was used, a larger analysis found that Strattera not only didn't worsen co-morbid tics, but seemed to improve them overall (Bloch 2009). Strattera also seems to be frequently effective in treating anxiety associated with ADHD (Tannock 2009, p.131).

- *Tenex* (guanfacine) and its once-a-day long-acting formulation *Intuniv*, and *Catapres* (clonidine) and its long-acting formulation *Kapvay*, are "alpha-2 agonists," which increase frontal lobe function. Like Strattera, they have no direct dopamine effect, either. The alpha-2 agonist medications seem to be most useful for impulsivity (as opposed to inattention). They are also utilized "off label" (without FDA approval for that indication) in the treatment of tics, and so are used frequently in Tourette's syndrome when tics and ADHD co-occur. Sedation and headaches are the most frequent complaints. Intuniv may be less sedating than Kapvay. Although the short-acting versions are also used as anti-hypertensive medications, they rarely cause any significant cardiovascular effects in our children. Keep children well hydrated, especially during the summer months. (A quick test of hydration status is the color of the child's urine: bright yellow is not adequate; almost clear white is the goal.) The school nurse may be asked to occasionally monitor the child's blood pressure and pulse. Alpha-2 agonists must be taken seven days per week and cannot be just stopped suddenly, as that that may cause dangerous rebound hypertension. Intuniv and Kapvay are also approved as "add-on" medications to the stimulants. Short-acting clonidine is also sometimes used at night to help insomnia in ADHD children.

- *Other medications* rarely used now for ADHD include Wellbutrin (bupropion) and tricyclic antidepressants (see section below on depression).

Comparative effectiveness of different ADHD treatments

In order to compare the relative effectiveness of different kinds of treatments across multiple studies, we need some statistics. Don't panic. This won't hurt a bit. What you need to know is the following. "Effect size" is a statistical tool that allows multiple studies—that were done perhaps using different scales/tests of effectiveness—to be compared with each other. An "effect size" of:

- 0.8 or greater is large (moves a patient from 50% to 79%)

- 0.5 is medium (moves a patient from 50% to 69%)

- 0.2 is small (moves a patient from 50% to 59%).

Table 14.1 shows how the different treatments for ADHD line up in terms of "effect size."

TABLE 14.1: Summary of effect sizes of different ADHD treatments (data from Barkley 2012 unless otherwise indicated)

Treatment	Effect size
Amphetamines (Adderall, Vyvanse, etc.)	1.0
Methylphenidate (Ritalin, Concerta, etc.)	0.75 (large effect size)
Atomoxetine (Strattera)	0.59
Intuniv	0.5 (medium effect size)
Omega-3 oil (Bloch and Qawasmi 2011)	0.31
Behavioral parent training	0.25–0.3
Neurofeedback (Hodgeson 2012)	0.21 (small effect size)

Medications for depression

Current research attributes biochemical depression to insufficient release by the brainstem of two neurotransmitters onto the cortex: serotonin and norepinephrine. Pharmacological treatments are thus aimed at raising the levels of these transmitters. The mainstays of antidepressants are the selective serotonin reuptake inhibitors (SSRIs).

In children, adolescents, and young adults, there appears to be small but real relationship of all antidepressants to increasing suicidal issues. This concern includes, but is not limited to, the SSRIs, and exists even if the "antidepressants" are being used for indications other than depression, such as for anxiety. Anticonvulsants are also associated with a small risk of suicidal issues for patients of all ages, no matter whether they are being used for neurobehavioral issues or for seizures. The periods of presumed greatest risk are with starting, increasing, or tapering of the medications. It is fair to say that more research will be helpful, and that any child, whether on antidepressant or anticonvulsant medication or not, should be carefully monitored for changes in behavior or ideation of self-harm. Updates can be found at www. fda.gov.

SSRIs (selective serotonin reuptake inhibitors)

SSRI medications selectively increase brain levels of serotonin by blocking its removal from the synapse between connecting neurons. More serotonin; less depression. Other drugs in the past have increased serotonin levels, but have not been selective about it, i.e., have raised other transmitter levels as well. Those additional undesirable transmitter levels have caused undesirable side effects.

The big fuss about SSRIs, then, is that their selectivity allows us to use highly effective doses on serotonin levels with fewer unpleasant side effects from other neurotransmitters. The SSRIs are usually medically quite safe, but some people may experience some unwelcome side effects.

The most common SSRI side effects are:

- weight gain

- sedation or insomnia

- sexual dysfunction

- occasional "dysinhibition," when the child gets more activated or agitated

- provocation of mania—this presents a thorny issue when impending bipolar first presents with a major depressive spell

- provocation of suicidal issues uncommonly as above

- cardiac effects: some antidepressants—Celexa (citalopram), Lexapro (escitalopram) and Elavil (amitriptyline)—have a "modest" prolongation effect on the heart's QT interval, perhaps making it prone to very serious arrhythmias. This effect seems to increase with higher dosages, and should be discussed with your doctor

- possible increased risk of bleeding or bruising, especially if taken with other medications with blood-thinning properties

- a rare, serious, emergency condition called "serotonin syndrome," marked by:

  ◦ mental status symptoms (such as agitation, hallucinations, or coma)

  ◦ vascular symptoms (such as rapid pulse, unstable blood pressure, fever, flushing, sweating, or dizziness)

  ◦ neuromuscular symptoms (such as tremor, stiffness, muscle jerks, increased reflexes, poor coordination, or seizures) and/or

  ◦ gastrointestinal symptoms (such as nausea, vomiting, or diarrhea).

SSRIs may take up to four to six weeks to become effective, unlike the stimulants that work within the hour. The class of SSRIs include:

- *Prozac* (fluoxetine): Prozac has been proven to help depression in about two-thirds of children. This is one of the few antidepressants that actually has approval for use in pediatric depression from the FDA. The doctor, though, may recommend other antidepressants. Other SSRIs include:

  ◦ *Zoloft* (sertraline)

  ◦ *Luvox* (fluvoxamine)—the brand "Luvox" is no longer manufactured

  ◦ *Paxil* (paroxetine)

  ◦ *Celexa* (citalopram)

  ◦ *Lexapro* (escitalopram—the active half of citalopram).

Other antidepressants

- *Wellbutrin* (bupropion) has been used with some apparent success for childhood depression as well as ADHD.

- *Effexor* (venlafaxine) is not currently recommended for use in children.

- *Elavil* (amitriptyline) and other traditional tricyclic antidepressants have been shown to be *ineffective* for depression in children and adolescents.

Medications for anxiety

See above warning regarding suicidal issues and antidepressants, which would apply to the use of antidepressants in children and young adults who are even being treated for reasons other than depression—such as for anxiety or OCD.

SSRIs

SSRIs are again the mainstay of medical treatment for anxiety, providing moderate or marked improvement in the majority of children with anxiety disorder. SSRIs are discussed further in the section above on medications for depression.

Other medications

Tricyclic antidepressant medications

Tricyclic medications are very effective for panic attacks, and many of them are quite helpful for anxiety in general. Their name derives from a chemical structure with three cyclic rings, hence "tricyclic."

The tricyclic medications tend to increase levels of multiple neurotransmitters (in contrast to the "selective" serotonin reuptake inhibitors). The tricyclics increase levels of serotonin and norepinephrine, but also affect histamine and cholinergic receptors.

The common side effects of the tricyclics are:

- sedation (a frequently significant problem)

- lightheadedness

- dry mouth

- constipation

- urinary retention

- rare, but potentially serious, cardiac effects, which have tempered their use, and may require monitoring with ECGs and blood drug levels.

Current tricyclic medications include:

- *Pamelor* (nortriptyline)

- *Tofranil* (imipramine)

- *Elavil* (amitriptyline).

Benzodiazepine anti-anxiety medications

The benzodiazepines raise levels of the transmitter GABA (gamma-aminobutyric acid). Although these medications have few serious systemic effects, they tend to be sedating, and require increasing doses over time. A significant potential exists for dependency on these medications. They are best used for just a short time, while waiting for the other medications to take effect. Like many other psychoactive medications, when they are no longer needed, their dose is typically slowly tapered. Commonly used benzodiazepines include:

- *Valium* (diazepam)

- *Klonopin* (clonazepam)

- *Ativan* (lorazepam)

- *Xanax* (alprazolam), which has a particularly short time of effectiveness, leading to frequent problematic rebound anxiety later in the day.

Buspar (buspirone)

Buspar may be effective for anxiety but not panic attacks. There are few serious medical side effects. It is not used as commonly as the SSRIs.

Medications for OCD

SSRIs are the mainstay of medical treatment for OCD. Not all of the SSRIs that are commonly used actually have current FDA approval for treatment of OCD in children. Overall, there appears to be a 40% reduction of symptoms (Freeman *et al.* 2004). See important information about the SSRIs in the section above on medications for depression.

Medications for bipolar disorder

Appropriate medication treatment of bipolar disorder is a work in progress. Recommendations depend in part on what stage is being treated (manic episode, depressive episode, or maintenance). Controlled data with large sample size is still frustratingly limited and conflicting (Goldstein 2012). Following are some of the medications that have been tried in bipolar disorder. Specific recommendations are debated, need to be individualized, and are beyond the scope of this text. Emerging evidence points to a potential role for omega-3 fatty acids in the treatment of mood disorders (Strawn *et al.* 2013).

Anticonvulsants

Anticonvulsants are commonly used as "mood stabilizers." These medications may require blood tests for drug levels, complete blood count, and liver function. In general, they are well tolerated. Possible side effects include:

- sedation

- weight gain (particularly Depakote)

- rare effects on the bone marrow, blood chemistries, or liver

- allergic reactions of the skin, eye, or mouth, which can be severe

- uncommon induction of suicidal issues has led to warnings for the entire class of anticonvulsants.

Anticonvulsants that have been used in bipolar disorder include:

- *Depakote* (sodium valproate)

- *Lamictal* (lamotrigine)

- *Tegretol* (carbamazepine).

Lithium

- *Lithium* is a complicated medication to use and has an unclear role in childhood bipolar disorder. Further, hopefully definitive research is pending.

Neuroleptics

Neuroleptics appear useful in bipolar disorder, especially for the psychotic and aggressive symptoms. Common neuroleptics include:

- *Risperdal* (risperidone)

- *Abilify* (aripiprazole)

- *Zyprexa* (olanzepine)

- *Haldol* (haloperidal)—no longer manufactured under the trade name Haldol

- *Orap* (pimozide)—used less commonly because of drug interactions and cardiac effects.

Risperdal, Abilify, and Zyprexa are examples of "atypical neuroleptics" because they have somewhat different side effect profiles than the older neuroleptics such as Haldol and Orap. Regardless, there are still significant possible side effects of this powerful class of medications. All of their potential long-term problems have not been fully determined yet. Some of the more common or important known side effects include:

- weight gain

- possible effects on blood sugar, including possibly inducing diabetes

- possible effects on other metabolic functions including lipid (cholesterol, etc.) changes

- possible effects on hormones including prolactin

- sedation

- effects on muscle control such as tremor or muscle rigidity

- a rare movement disorder called "tardive dyskinesia," which is particularly rare in children with the newer atypical neuroleptics, but may be permanent

- a rare but dangerous metabolic condition of high fever, muscle destruction, and confusion called "malignant neuroleptic syndrome"

- neuroleptics carry a warning of increased suicidality

- difficulty swallowing

- rare prolonged erection, which is a medical emergency if lasting more than four hours

- cardiac effects, which are not commonly significant with many of the neuroleptics

- rare effects on the complete blood count (CBC).

In patients with diagnoses of both bipolar depression and co-morbid ADHD, it is important to first stabilize the mood using agents such as the above before attempting to treat the ADHD—in order to decrease the risk of inducing a manic spell. Routine anti-depressants can also trigger a manic spell.

Medications for tic disorders

The relative efficacy of medications for tics is summarized as follows:

- Risperdal (risperidone), Abilify (aripiprazole), Haldol (haloperidol), Orap (pimozide) have good evidence with 35–65% tic reduction (Wu 2010).

- Catapres (clonidine) and Tenex (guanfacine) show modest efficacy for tic reduction at 25% and 30% respectively (Wu 2010).

- Strattera (atomoxetine) showed 25% tic reduction in patients with ADHD and tics (Wu 2010).

- Omega-3 fatty acids have been shown ineffective for actual tic severity per se, but showed improvement in quality of life scores (Gabbay 2012).

Despite being somewhat less effective, the alpha-2 agonists such as Catapres (clonidine) and Tenex (guanfacine) may frequently be tried first given their relative safety profile compared to neuroleptics. Note that only the neuroleptics Haldol and Orap have actual FDA approval for use in tics; and Orap is rarely used now because of drug interactions and severe potential cardiac arrhythmias. More information on these medications can be found in the sections on medications for bipolar disorder and ADHD.

Medications used in the autism spectrum disorders (ASDs)

Unfortunately, there are currently no FDA approved medications for the core socialization/communication/repetitive problems of children with an ASD. Medications can be somewhat helpful, though, for the co-morbidities that frequently accompany the ASD. Children on the spectrum typically show less effectiveness and more side effects to medications in general than "neurotypical" children, and tend to require lower medication doses. The available evidence of medication use in ASD was summarized by Mohiuddin (2012).

- Risperdal (risperidone) and Abilify (aripiprazole) are approved for irritability in 6–17-year-olds with autistic disorder.

- SSRIs such as Prozac (see above) are probably ineffective when used for repetitive behaviors, but still might be useful for anxiety in spectrum children. Kids with ASD are very sensitive to the SSRIs and require low doses.

- Stimulants, Strattera (atomoxetine), and Catapres (clonidine) all treat hyperactivity.

- Methylphenidate compounds such as Ritalin appear helpful in treating aggression.

The topic of Complementary and Alternative Treatments (CATs) for the ASDs is filled with controversy. Suffice it to say here that most "traditional" authorities feel that such treatments are in general without sufficient evidence of effectiveness to merit recommendation, and several can be harmful. According to the American Academy of Pediatrics (AAP 2013), "Few CAM treatments have been sufficiently studied to permit evidence-based endorsement of their use. Of the few that have been studied, most have been found to be ineffective." In addition, such treatments can divert time and financial resources from other approaches that do have good evidence of effectiveness. Just because a treatment has not been approved by the FDA for effectiveness or safety, this doesn't necessarily make it a good idea! Be leery about approaches that are offered without peer review publication of studies that employed effective blinding of the participants/raters and utilized comparison to a control group that didn't receive the treatment. If using a CAT, be sure to set clear goals regarding target symptoms and carefully monitor the progress/effectiveness of the intervention. Having said all of that, it's been pointed out that lack of proof doesn't necessarily mean that a treatment doesn't work—just, perhaps, that it is yet to be proven. Also, some treatments may address exacerbating issues, such as avoiding dairy if the child also has a milk allergy, or treating a child's constipation.

For more details, see the website of the Association for Science in Autism Treatment at www.asatonline.org. For even more, heavy duty detailed information, see the article "A Review of Complementary and Alternative Treatments for Autism Spectrum Disorders" (Lofthouse *et al.* 2012).

Behavioral Checklist

Child's name: Your name:

Date: Subject (if teacher):

Please rate the severity of each problem listed, and add comments in the margins as needed.

0 = none   1 = slight   2 = moderate   3 = major

	0	1	2	3
Easily distracted	☐	☐	☐	☐
Requires one-to-one attention to get work done	☐	☐	☐	☐
Impulsive (trouble waiting turn, blurts out answers)	☐	☐	☐	☐
Hyperactive (fidgety, trouble staying seated)	☐	☐	☐	☐
Disorganized	☐	☐	☐	☐
Does not write down assignments	☐	☐	☐	☐
Backpack is a mess	☐	☐	☐	☐
Poor sense of time	☐	☐	☐	☐
Over-reacts	☐	☐	☐	☐
Easily overwhelmed	☐	☐	☐	☐
Blows up easily	☐	☐	☐	☐

Trouble switching activities	☐	☐	☐	☐
Poor handwriting	☐	☐	☐	☐
Certain academic tasks seem difficult (specify)	☐	☐	☐	☐
Anxious, edgy, stressed, or painfully worried	☐	☐	☐	☐
Obsessive thoughts or fears; perseverative rituals	☐	☐	☐	☐
Seems *deliberately* spiteful, cruel, or annoying	☐	☐	☐	☐
Irritated for hours or days on end (not just frequent, brief blow-ups)	☐	☐	☐	☐
Depressed, "empty," sad, or unhappy; loss of interests	☐	☐	☐	☐
Extensive mood swings	☐	☐	☐	☐
Tics: repetitive movements or noises	☐	☐	☐	☐
Poor eye contact	☐	☐	☐	☐
Does not catch on to social cues	☐	☐	☐	☐
Limited range of interests and interactions	☐	☐	☐	☐
Unusual sensitivity to sounds, touch, textures, movement, or taste	☐	☐	☐	☐
Coordination difficulties	☐	☐	☐	☐
Other (specify)	☐	☐	☐	☐

If the child is on medication, please answer the following questions:

Can you tell when the child is on medication or not?

Does the medication work consistently throughout the day?

Does the child appear to be on too much or too little medication?

Other comments:

Quick Quiz on Executive Function

Answer the questions below based on the following scenario.

> John is a bright, college-bound eighth grade student with ADHD (attention deficit hyperactivity disorder). He does not write down a required essay into his assignment pad, and does not hand in the required work. His teacher tells him that if he simply hands in the essay tomorrow, it will still receive full credit.
>
> This time, the teacher watches John write down the assignment on a slip of paper. John thanks the teacher, truly intends to do it, walks into the hall and throws the slip into his backpack. When he arrives home, his mother asks him about his homework, but the subject of the essay never comes up. John never does hand it in. The teacher gives John a zero, hoping that it will teach him a lesson for next time.

1. John primarily hurts himself by this behavior.

   a. True

   b. False

2. There are logical reasons why people would choose to "shoot themselves in their own foot."

   a. True

   b. False

3. Instead, problems with executive function could explain this behavior.

   a. True

   b. False

4. Organization problems are common in ADHD.

   a. True

   b. False

5. John comes home, finds the note, and yet never tells his mother. This can be best explained by:

   a. John is lazy, and yet somehow musters enough energy to deliberately sabotage his own future.

   b. John wants to deceive his mother, even though he has been granted "amnesty" if he just hands in the essay.

   c. John lives in the next four seconds. For the next four seconds, the most appealing choice is to ignore the problem.

6. This teacher has already gone above and beyond typical understanding and guidance.

   a. True

   b. False

7. The purpose of giving John a "zero" is to:

   a. Cause him to squirm.

   b. Alter his behavior next time.

8. For people with ADHD, there is no "next time."

   a. True

   b. False

9. Giving John a "zero" is likely to alter his ADHD behavior next time.

   a. True

   b. False

10. If a strategy doesn't work, it makes sense to:

    a. Keep repeating it, hoping the 53rd time will be the charm.

    b. Try something else.

11. The reason why John doesn't act like everyone else is that:

    a. He *can't* consistently act like everyone else.

    b. He likes getting yelled at.

12. Entrusting a child who has executive function problems with his own organization and future planning is a good idea.

    a. True

    b. False

13. Direct communication between the teacher and the parent or skills teacher is more likely to be a successful intervention.

    a. True

    b. False

14. Most children shouldn't need this type of continuous support. It's "weird" that John does. That is why he has a diagnosable condition.

    a. True

    b. False

15. This all makes sense during this quiz. The next time I encounter such a situation in the real world, I will...

Answers should be self-evident.

Dealing with Insomnia

Sleep Hygiene

Insomnia is a prominent component of many conditions of the syndrome mix, including ADHD, anxiety, and depression. Discuss sleep problems with your doctor, as the differential diagnosis also includes such medical conditions as obstructive sleep apnea and restless leg syndrome. Some sleep problems require consultation with a sleep specialist, who may recommend an overnight "sleep study."

Treatment recommendations for most types of insomnia include "sleep hygiene."

Sleep hygiene is a full day issue.

- Regulate time and amount of sleep.

    ○ Ensure a consistent time of awakening and of bedtime (no more than one-hour variation on non-school days compared with school days).

    ○ Ensure a consistent amount of sleep (for children 6–10 years old, about 10.5 hours; for children 10–17 years old, about 9 hours).

    ○ No naps post preschool age (napping post preschool age is a sign of sleep deprivation, as are trouble waking up in the morning, and sleeping later on non-school days).

- Regulate the environment *before* bedtime.

    ○ No electronics or exciting or stressful activities for at least one hour before bedtime. (That includes no stressful homework. There should not be a television in the child's bedroom.)

- ◦ No exercise for one to four hours before bed (although exercise earlier during the day is important for sleep and general health).

- ◦ No big meals right before bed (may have to allow late food for children with poor appetite during the day).

- ◦ No caffeinated drinks (including sodas) in the evening.

- ◦ Do have a consistent, calming bedtime routine.

- ◦ Do keep the home positive and on a regular schedule.

- Regulate environment *at* bedtime.

  - ◦ A child's bed should be used only for sleeping, i.e., no reading in bed, and certainly no electronics. The goal is to condition the child that when he gets into bed, then he falls asleep. Some doctors suggest getting out of bed if you haven't fallen asleep within half an hour and doing a calming activity (no electronics) until tired, and then returning to bed.

  - ◦ The child should fall asleep independently in his own bed, and not in his parents' room. A mind-calming activity such as a simple meditation technique may be helpful. See www.pediatricneurology.com/stress.htm for an easy deep breathing/muscle relaxation meditation exercise.

  - ◦ Room should be cool, quiet, dark at night (a nightlight is okay) and bright in the morning.

If sleep hygiene is insufficient to handle the insomnia, then medications such as melatonin or clonidine should be discussed with your doctor. Note that melatonin should be given two to four hours before desired sleep time.

Further Reading

Views of the following resources do not necessarily represent the views of the authors.

General neurobehavioral information

Books

Brown, T. E. (ed.) (2009) *ADHD Comorbidities: Handbook for ADHD Complications in Children and Adults.* Arlington, VA: American Psychiatric Publishing, Inc.

Presents an encyclopedic review of the literature on drug and behavioral treatments. Intended for professional use.

Dulcan, M.K. (ed.) (2009) *Textbook of Child and Adolescent Psychiatry.* Arlington, VA: American Psychiatric Publishing.

This is a professional level textbook.

Ratey, J. and Johnson, C. (1998) *Shadow Syndromes.* New York: Bantam Books.

This book explains that many symptoms such as attention deficit hyperactivity disorder (ADHD), obsessions, rage, autism, etc. can occur at "subsyndromal" levels. Human brains are not "all or nothing."

Shore, K. (2002) *Special Kids Problem Solver: Ready-to-Use Interventions for Helping All Students with Academic, Behavioral and Physical Problems.* San Francisco, CA: Jossey-Bass.

The title is says it all.

Internet resources

www.pediatricneurology.com is the author's website, featuring detailed information and links on most of the conditions covered in this book, as well as other pediatric neurological issues such as headaches and seizures.

National Institutes of Health at www.nlm.nih.gov/medlineplus covers a wide range of neurobehavioral disorders in depth.

See **http://iacapap.org/iacapap-textbook-of-child-and-adolescent-mental-health** for a free international textbook online on child and adolescent mental health.

Dr. Ross Greene's site www.livesinthebalance.org gives detailed, thoughtful, and empathic information about the collaborative problem-solving approach, which is described briefly in Chapter 2 of this book, and can be useful with most conditions of the syndrome mix.

Pediatric Psychiatry Pamphlets at http://jamesdauntchandler.tripod.com by Dr. Jim Chandler provide good-natured, accessible, concise, responsible information on a large variety of conditions including ADHD, oppositional defiant disorder (ODD), obsessive-compulsive disorder (OCD), tics, panic, and bipolar disorders.

www.addwarehouse.com carries a full selection of books for teachers and parents on the whole spectrum of neurobehavioral disorders, not just ADHD.

The National Alliance on Mental Illness at www.nami.org covers a large assortment of neurobehavioral disorders.

www.childmind.org has useful information on a variety of childhood neurobehavioral issues. Subscribe to their newsletter at http://support.childmind. org/site/PageNavigator/forms/subscribe_full.html.

www.commonsensemedia.org previews computer programs/websites/apps for children.

Internet sites dedicated to medications

www.drugs.com covers all medications with information for the general public and also at the professional level. See also their drug interaction checker and pill identifier resources.

www.parentsmedguide.org contains fantastic guides focused on the medication treatments of ADHD, depression, and bipolar. Prepared jointly by the American Psychiatric Association and the American Academy of Child and Adolescent Psychiatry.

www.fda.gov posts updates on medication emanating from the US Food and Drug Administration.

Attention deficit hyperactivity disorder (ADHD)

Books

Barkley, R. (2005) *ADHD and the Nature of Self Control*. New York: Guilford Press.

More on the theory of ADHD, with some excellent practical advice. Fairly advanced reading.

Barkley, R. (2005) *Attention-Deficit Hyperactive Disorder: A Handbook for Diagnosis and Treatment* (3rd edition). New York: Guilford Press.

The scientific and unbelievably extensive literature review of ADHD underlying Dr. Barkley's concepts. Like most medical "handbooks," it barely fits in your hand. Quite advanced reading.

Barkley, R. (2013) *Taking Charge of ADHD*. New York: Guilford Press.

Dr. Barkley offers ground-breaking material on the nature of ADHD and executive functions. Harder, less optimistic reading designed primarily for parents.

Brown, T.E. (2013) *A New Understanding of ADHD in Children and Adults: Executive Function Impairments*. New York: Routledge.

Scientific yet highly readable book on executive function and ADHD by a leading researcher in the area.

Green, C. and Chee, K. (1997) *Understanding ADHD*. New York: Vermilion.

This book addresses serious issues in an upbeat, even funny, style. A great place to start reading.

Hallowell, E.M. and Jensen, P.S. (2010) *Superparenting for ADHD: An Innovative Approach to Raising Your Distracted Child*. New York: Ballantine.

Two leaders in the field put together a wonderful, optimistic book stressing the positive aspects of life with ADHD.

Hallowell, E.M. and Ratey, J.R. (2011) *Driven to Distraction*. New York: Simon and Schuster.

This excellent book about ADHD has become the standard starting point, especially for adults with ADHD. Many parents might find themselves in this book.

Hoopman, K. (2008) *All Dogs Have ADHD*. London: Jessica Kingsley Publishers.

An incredibly adorable book using photos of dogs to enhance the "right on" captions, which playfully explain the symptoms of ADHD to children (and adults). See the companion book, *All Cats Have Asperger Syndromes*.

Kutscher, M.L. (2003) *ADHD Book: Living Right Now!* New York: Neurology Press.

The author's first complete, succinct book on the extended range of ADHD problems and treatments. Realistic but upbeat.

Kutscher, M.L. (2009) *ADHD—Living without Brakes*. London: Jessica Kingsley Publishers.

The author's updated book on ADHD emphasizing executive function and co-morbidity aspects. Treatment is based on four principles.

1. Keep it positive.

2. Keep it calm.

3. Keep it organized.

4. Keep doing points one to three.

Kutscher M.L. and Moran, M. (2009) *Organizing the Disorganized Child: Simple Strategies to Succeed in School*. New York: Harper Collins.

Practical approaches to teach your child how to be organized, and how to effectively read, write, and study.

Laurie, T.E. and Quinn, P.O. (2010) *Ready for Take-Off: Preparing Your Teen with ADHD or LD for College*. Maryland, MD: Magination Press.

Uses the high school years to teach your teen the academic and daily life skills that they will need in college.

Pera, G. (2008) *Is It You, Me, or Adult A.D.D.? Stopping the Roller Coaster when Someone You Love Has Attention Deficit Disorder.* San Francisco, CA: 1201 Alarm Press.

Wonderful reading if you or your spouse has ADHD.

Phelan, T.W. (2000) *All about Attention Deficit Disorder.* Glen Ellyn, IL: Child Management Press.

All about ADHD for parents and teachers. Like all of his excellent books on childhood behavior, this book is both very useful and actually fun to read.

Phelan, T.W. (2012) *Surviving Your Adolescents: How to Manage and Let Go of Your 13–18 Year Olds.* Glen Ellyn, IL: Child Management Press.

Particularly useful for ADHD adolescents, who have a double dose of foresight blindness. Especially encouraging for ADHDer parents, because this book describes how many families of typical teenagers experience difficulty similar to their ADHD teen—and most of them seem to turn into typical adults.

Zeigler Dendy, C.A. (2006) *Teenagers with ADD: A Guide for Parents.* Bethesda, MD: Woodbine House.

Optimistic and practical advice for teenagers and others with ADHD. It features extensive sections on specific problems such as waking up and organization. There are also extensive lists of school (and home) accommodations.

Internet resources

CHADD (Children and Adults with Attention Deficit/Hyperactivity Disorders) at www.chadd.org is an excellent, all-inclusive support group with local chapters. Phone: (001) 800-233-4050.

National Resource Center for ADHD (a project of CHADD) at www.help4adhd.org has terrific, balanced information on ADHD. They have information specialists available online or at (001) 800-233-4050.

www.parentsmedguide.org contains fantastic guides about the diagnosis and medical treatments of ADHD, depression, and bipolar. Prepared by the American Psychiatric Association and the American Academy of Child and Adolescent Psychiatry.

www.addresources.org has a multitude of free articles on ADHD in children and adults, with more readings available to members.

Center for ADHD Awareness, Canada at www.caddac.ca provides a wide variety of useful material especially targeted to Canadian readers.

www.addvance.com specializes particularly in girls and women with ADHD, as well as college issues in their "Help for Young Adults" section. They offer a wide range of excellent books. In particular, see their books *Understanding Girls with ADHD* and *Putting on the Brakes.*

ADDitude Magazine at www.additudemag.com is an electronic version of their excellent print magazine on ADHD.

Links on developing an IEP (Individual Educational Plan) at **www.teach-nology.com/teachers/special_ed/iep.**

Teens with ADHD site and book by Chris Dendy at **www.chrisdendy.com.**

Internet email newsletters (excellent for reminding yourself of ADHD principles of care)

www.helpforadd.com by Dr. David Rabiner is a very useful and scientifically sound email newsletter.

www.childmind.org emails a newsletter on a variety of children's neurobehavioral problems. Sign up at http://support.childmind.org/site/PageNavigator/forms/subscribe_full.html.

Learning disabilities (LDs)

Books

Osman, B.B. (1997) *Learning Disabilities and ADHD: A Family Guide to Living and Learning Together.* New York: Wiley.

Shaywitz, S. (2003) *Overcoming Dyslexia: A New and Complete Science-Based Program for Overcoming Reading Problems at Any Level.* New York: Vintage.

Internet resources

LD Online at www.ldonline.org is a superb resource including fair, full text, useful articles. Spend an evening there! Includes ADHD, writing, learning, speech, and social difficulties. For suggestions on books for kids to read about LD, see www.ldonline.org/kids/books.

National Center for Learning Disabilities at www.ncld.org is another great source of information on a wide variety of learning disabilities. The material is well organized.

International Dyslexia Association at www.interdys.org has excellent, well-organized material with international resources.

Smart Kids with LD at www.smartkidswithld.org has well-organized material explaining learning disabilities with an eye towards a child's legal rights.

Asperger's syndrome

Books

General

Attwood, T. (1998) *Asperger's Syndrome: A Guide for Parents and Professionals.* London: Jessica Kingsley Publishers.

An excellent (brief) diagnostic and treatment resource. See the author's website at *www.tonyattwood.com.au,* which includes numerous excellent articles and an Asperger's rating scale.

Attwood, T. (2007) *The Complete Guide to Asperger's Syndrome.* London: Jessica Kingsley Publishers.

A comprehensive book from a leader in the field.

Bashe, P. and Kirby, B. (2005) *The OASIS Guide to Asperger Syndrome.* New York: Crown Publishers.

Another excellent and complete resource (lengthy), written empathically and fairly.

Brady, L.J. (2011) *Apps for Autism: A Must-Have Resource for the Special Needs Community.* Arlington, TX: Future Horizons.

Independent reviews of hundreds of apps.

Hoopman, K. (2006) *All Cats Have Asperger Syndrome.* London: Jessica Kingsley Publishers.

An incredibly adorable book using photos of cats to enhance the "right on" captions, which playfully explain the symptoms of Asperger's to children (and adults). See the companion book, *All Dogs Have ADHD.*

Jackson, L. (2002) *Freaks, Geeks, and Asperger Syndrome: A User Guide to Adolescence.* London: Jessica Kingsley Publishers.

Filled with understanding and advice from a teen with Asperger's.

Volkmar, F.R. and Wiesner, L.A. (2009) *A Practical Guide to Autism: What Every Parent, Family Member and Teacher Needs to Know.* Hoboken, NJ: John Wiley and Sons.

A comprehensive, easy to read guide to everything you need to know in order to navigate your child through your and his new world.

Willey, L.H. (1999) *Pretending to be Normal: Living with Asperger's Syndrome.* London: Jessica Kingsley Publishers.

A powerful, elegant autobiography that traces the struggles faced by children and adults with Asperger's. Several appendices provide practical advice for students, employees, and parents.

Asperger's and friendship

Cook O'Toole, J. (2013) *The Asperkid's Secret Book of Social Rules.* London: Jessica Kingsley Publishers.

Dubin, N. (2007) *Asperger Syndrome and Bullying: Strategies and Solutions.* London: Jessica Kingsley Publishers.

Gray, C. (2006) *No Fishing Allowed: "Reel" In Bullying.* Arlington, TX: Future Horizons.

Gray, C. (2010) *The New Social Story Book.* Arlington, TX: Future Horizons.

Heinrichs, R. (2003) *Perfect Targets: Asperger Syndrome and Bullying.* Kansas: Autism Asperger Publishing Company.

Schneider, C. (2007) *Acting Antics: A Theatrical Approach to Teaching Social Understanding to Kids and Teens with Asperger Syndrome.* London: Jessica Kingsley Publishers.

The Secret Agent Society www.sst-institute.net.

Williams White, S. (2011) *Social Skills Training for Children with Asperger Syndrome and High-Functioning Autism.* New York: The Guilford Press.

Asperger's and CBT

Attwood, T. (2004) *Exploring Feelings: Cognitive Behaviour Therapy to Manage Anger.* Arlington, TX: Future Horizons.

Attwood, T. and Garnett, M. (2013) *CBT to Help Young People with Asperger's Syndrome to Understand and Express Affection*. London: Jessica Kingsley Publishers.

Callesen, K., Moller-Nielsen, A. and Attwood, T. (2008) *CAT-kit*. Arlington, TX: Future Horizons.

Mind Reading: The Interactive Guide to Emotions. Interactive DVD distributed by Jessica Kingsley Publishers, London.

Scarpa, A., Wells, A. and Attwood, T. (2013) *Exploring Feelings for Young Children with High-Functioning Autism or Asperger's Disorder*. London: Jessica Kingsley Publishers.

Scarpa A., Williams White, S. and Attwood, T. (eds) (2013) *CBT for Children and Adolescents with High-Functioning Autism Spectrum Disorder*. New York: The Guilford Press.

Internet resources

www.autismspeaks.org has everything you could ask for from a website, presenting open-minded but research-based information. In particular, see their tool kits such as the "100 day kit" for families of newly diagnosed children, and their selection of apps rated by degree of scientific validation.

Jessica Kingsley Publishers website at www.jkp.com has an unbelievable selection of books on the autism spectrum and related conditions.

Future Horizons at http://fhautism.com specializes in autism spectrum and sensory needs children.

Sign up for an excellent parent oriented magazine **Autism/Asperger's Digest at http://autismdigest.com**.

www.tonyattwood.com.au is Dr. Attwood's informative website.

www.cat-kit.com features Dr. Attwood's Cognitive Affective Training kit.

www.nldontheweb.org has excellent information on non-verbal learning disabilities.

See the website of the **Association for Science in Autism Treatment at www.asatonline.org** for non-biased information about traditional and non-traditional treatments.

For even more, heavy duty detailed information on Complementary and Alternative Treatments by Lofthouse, N., Hendren, R., Hurt, E., Arnold, L.E. and Butter, E. (2012) see the article **"A Review of Complementary and Alternative Treatments for Autism Spectrum Disorders"** (website address is **www.hindawi.com/journals/aurt/2012/870391**). Last accessed December 2013.

www.awaare.org is dedicated to educating everyone about the risks of spectrum children "taking off," with particular emphasis on preventing drowning.

Anxiety/OCD

Internet resources

Anxiety and Depression Association of America at www.adaa.org covers the whole spectrum of anxiety disorders.

International OCD Foundation at www.ocfoundation.org has terrific information on OCD. Includes pages appropriate for reading by different age groups.

Sensory integration dysfunction

Books

Dalgliesh, C. (2013) *The Sensory Child Gets Organized.* New York: Touchstone Books.

> This book covers sensory symptoms that accompany a wide variety of conditions. Useful parenting and organizing tips.

Kranowitz, C.S. and Miller, L.J. (2005) *The Out-of-Sync Child: Recognizing and Coping with Sensory Integration Dysfunction.* New York: Skylight Press.

> This wonderful book covers the diagnosis and treatment of sensory integration dysfunction. Makes sense out of a very broad topic.

Internet resource

Sensory Processing Disorder Foundation at www.spdfoundation.net has information and a store online for sensory needs supplies.

Tourette's syndrome

Book

Dornbush, M. and Pruitt, S. (1995) *Teaching the Tiger.* California: Hope Press.

> This text is an entire book of accommodations for Tourette's students. Many of these ideas apply to ADHD and LD students as well.

Internet resources

Tourette Syndrome "Plus" at www.tourettesyndrome.net is an awesome and practical site on Tourette's, OCD, rage, etc. by Leslie E. Packer.

National Tourette Syndrome Association has great information and lists its local support group chapters at **www.tsa-usa.org**.

Bipolar disorder

Book

Papolos, D. (2006) *The Bipolar Child.* New York: Broadway Books.

> This is an excellent diagnostic and treatment resource. This book has brought awareness about bipolar disorder in children into the public realm.

Internet resources

www.thebalancedmind.org is a great site on bipolar disorder.

www.parentsmedguide.org contains fantastic guides about the diagnosis and medical treatments of ADHD, depression, and bipolar. Prepared by the American Psychiatric Association and the American Academy of Child and Adolescent Psychiatry.

Oppositional defiant disorder
Books

Barkley, R.A. and Benton, C.M. (2013) *Your Defiant Child: Eight Steps to Better Behavior.* New York: Guilford Press.

A book for caregivers of oppositional/defiant children who want to restore a loving relationship with their child.

Greene, R.W. (2010) *The Explosive Child: A New Approach for Understanding and Parenting Easily Frustrated, Chronically Inflexible Children.* New York: HarperCollins.

A must read for parents of inflexible-explosive children who do not respond well to typical reward systems—whether or not they have oppositional defiant disorder. This book is wonderfully and empathically written.

Central auditory processing disorders
Book

Bellis, T.J. (2003) *When the Brain Can't Hear: Unraveling the Mystery of Auditory Processing Disorders.* New York: Simon and Schuster.

Internet resources

A comprehensive article on CAPD by Dr. Donna Geffner and Eve Kessler is found at **www.smartkidswithld.org/ld-basics/treatments-and-support/central-auditory-processing-disorder**.

www.ldonline.org has information on CAPD in its section on "Processing Deficits."

American Speech-Language-Hearing Association at www.asha.org has CAPD information.

References

AACAP Practice Parameter (2012) "Practice parameter for evaluation and treatment of children and adolescents with suicidal behavior." *Journal of the American Academy of Child and Adolescent Psychiatry 40*, 7, Supplement, 24S–51S.

American Academy of Pediatrics (2012) "Sensory integration therapies for children with developmental and behavioral disorders." *Pediatrics 129*, 6, 1186.

American Academy of Pediatrics (2013) "Complementary and Alternative Medication Therapies." In *Autism: Caring for Children with ASDs: A Toolkit for Clinicians* (2nd edition). Elk Grove Village, IL: American Academy of Pediatrics.

APA (American Psychiatric Association) (1994) *Diagnostic and Statistical Manual of Mental Disorders-IV.* Washington, DC: American Psychiatric Association.

APA (American Psychiatric Association) (2013) *Diagnostic and Statistical Manual of Mental Disorders-5.* Washington, DC: American Psychiatric Association.

Arnsten, A. (2005) "Neurobiology of executive functions: catecholamine influences on prefrontal cortical functions." *Biological Psychiatry 57*, 11, 1377–1384.

Bader, A. (2012) "Complementary and alternative medication in children and adolescents with ADHD." *Current Opinion Pediatrics 24*, 6, 760.

Baeyens, D. (2004) "ADHD in children with nocturnal eneuresis." *Journal of Urology 71*, 6 (part 2), 2576–2759.

Barkley, R. (1998) *Attention-Deficit Hyperactivity Disorder: A Handbook for Diagnosis and Treatment* (2nd edition). New York: Guilford Press.

Barkley, R. (2012) *ADHD Report.* October 2012. New York: Guilford Press.

Barkley, R. (2013) *Taking Charge of ADHD.* New York: Guilford Press.

Barkley, R.A., Fischer, M., Edelbrock, C. and Smallish, L. (1990) "The adolescent outcome of hyperactive children diagnosed by research criteria: an 8-year prospective follow-up study." *Journal of the American Academy of Child and Adolescent Psychiatry 29*, 546–557.

Beiderman, J. (2012) *25th European College of Neuropsychopharmacology Conference.* October 2012.

Biederman, J., Monuteaux, M.C., Mick, E., Spencer, T., Wilens, T.E., Silva, J.M., *et al.* (2006) "Young adult outcome of attention deficit hyperactivity disorder: a controlled 10-year follow-up study." *Psychological Medicine 36*, 2, 167–179.

Bernstein, G. and Layne, A. (2004) "Separation Anxiety Disorder and Generalized Anxiety Disorder." In J. Wiener and M. Dulcan (eds) *Textbook of Child and Adolescent Psychiatry* (3rd edition). Arlington, VA: American Psychiatric Publishing.

Bloch, M. (2009) "Meta-analysis: treatment of ADHD in children with comorbid tic disorder." *Journal of the American Academy of Child and Adolescent Psychiatry 48*, 884–893.

Bloch, M. and Qawasmi, A. (2011) "Omega-3 fatty acid supplementation for the treatment of children with attention-deficit/hyperactivity disorder symptomatology: systematic review and meta-analysis." *Journal of the American Academy of Child and Adolescent Psychiatry 50*, 10, 991–1000.

Brent, D.A. (2013) "Ending the silence on gun violence." *Journal of the American Academy of Child and Adolescent Psychiatry 52*, 4, 333–338.

Brooks, R. and Goldstein, S. (2001) *Raising Resilient Children.* New York: McGraw-Hill.

Brown, T. (2009) *ADHD Comorbidities: Handbook for ADHD Complications in Children and Adults.* Washington, DC: American Psychiatric Publishing, Inc.

Carver, J. (2005) "The Highway Patrol Approach to Discipline and Correction." Available at www.drjoecarver.com/clients/49355/File/The%20Highway%20 Patrol%20Approach%20to%20Discipline%20and%20Correction.html, accessed on December 23, 2013.

CDC (2012) *Suicide: Risk and Protective Factors.* Atlanta, GA: CDC. Available at www.cdc.gov/violenceprevention/suicide/riskprotectivefactors.html, accessed on November 13, 2013.

CDC (2013) "Mental health surveillance among children—United States, 2005–2011." *Morbidity and Mortality Weekly Report 62*, 2 Supplement.

Charach, A. (2013) "Interventions for preschool children at high risk for ADHD: a comparative effectiveness review." *Pediatrics 131*, 5, 1384.

Covey, S.R. (1989) *The Seven Habits of Highly Effective People: Restoring the Character Ethic.* New York: Simon and Schuster.

Feinstein, C. and Phillips, I. (2004) "Developmental Disorders of Learning, Motor Skills, and Communication." In J. Wiener and M. Dulcan (eds) *Textbook of Child and Adolescent Psychiatry* (3rd edition). Arlington, VA: American Psychiatric Publishing.

Florida Department of Education (2001) *Auditory Processing Disorders.* Technical Assistance Paper FY 2001-9. Tallahassee, FL: Florida Department of Education. Available at www.aitinstitute.org/CAPD_technical_assistance_paper.pdf, accessed on December 24, 2013.

Freeman, J.B., Garcia, A.M., Swedo, S.E., *et al.* (2004) "Obsessive-Compulsive Disorder." In J. Wiener and M. Dulcan (eds) *Textbook of Child and Adolescent Psychiatry* (3rd edition). Arlington, VA: American Psychiatric Publishing.

Gabbay, V. (2012) "A double blind, placebo controlled trial of omega-3 fatty acids in Tourette's Disorder." *Pediatrics 129*, 6, 1493.

Garnett, K. (1998) *Math Learning Disabilities.* Available at www.ldonline.org/article/5896, accessed January 5, 2014.

Goldstein, B. (2012) "Pharmacologic treatment of bipolar disorder in children and adolescents." *Child and Adolescent Psychiatric Clinics of North America 21*, 911–939.

Goldstein, B. (2013) "Do stimulants prevent substance use and misuse among youth with AD/HD? The answer is still maybe." *Journal of the American Academy of Child and Adolescent Psychiatry 52*, 3, 225–226.

Greene, R.W. (1999) *The Explosive Child: A New Approach for Understanding and Parenting Easily Frustrated, Chronically Inflexible Children.* London: HarperCollins.

Greene, R.W. (2010) *The Explosive Child: A New Approach for Understanding and Parenting Easily Frustrated, Chronically Inflexible Children.* London: HarperCollins.

Hallowell, E. and Jensen, P. (2008) *Super-parenting for ADD: An Innovative Approach to Raising Your Distracted Child.* New York: Ballantine Books.

Hammerness, P. (2011) "Cardiovascular risk of stimulant treatment of pediatric ADHD: update and clinical recommendations." *Journal of the American Academy of Child and Adolescent Psychiatry 50*, 10, 978.

Harris, E. and Wu, S. (2010) "Children with tic disorders: how to match treatment with symptoms." *Current Psychiatry 9*, 3, 29–36.

Hodgeson, K. (2012) "Nonpharmacological treatment for ADHD: a meta-analysis review." *Journal of Attention Disorders*, May 29.

Houston, A. (2013) "Groundbreaking report shows increases in children's psychiatric disorders." *Child and Adolescent Psychopharmacology Update 15*, 7, 7.

Jensen, P.S., Hinshaw, S.P., Swanson, J.M., Greenhill, L.L., Conners, C.K., Arnold, L.E., *et al.* (2001) "Findings from the NIMH Multimodal Treatment Study of ADHD (MTA); implications and applications for primary care providers." *Journal of Developmental and Behavioral Pediatrics 22*, 1, 60–73.

King, R. and Leckman, J. (2004) "Tic Disorders." In J. Wiener and M. Dulcan (eds) *Textbook of Child and Adolescent Psychiatry* (3rd edition). Arlington, VA: American Psychiatric Publishing.

Klein, R. (2012) "Clinical and functional outcome of childhood ADHD 33 years later." *Archives of General Psychiatry 69*, 12, 1295.

Kranowitz, C.S. (1998) *The Out-Of-Sync Child: Recognizing and Coping with Sensory Integration Dysfunction.* New York: Skylight Press.

Kranowitz, C.S. (2005) *The Out-Of-Sync Child: Recognizing and Coping with Sensory Integration Dysfunction.* New York: Skylight Press.

Kutscher, M.L. (2009) *ADHD—Living without Brakes.* London: Jessica Kingsley Publishers.

Kutscher, M.L. and Moran, M. (2009) *Organizing the Disorganized Child: Simple Strategies to Succeed in School.* New York: HarperCollins.

Larson, K., Russ, S., Kahn, R. and Halfon, N. (2011) "Patterns of comorbidity, functioning, and service use for US children with ADHD, 2007." *Pediatrics 127*, 3, 462–470.

Lecendreux, M. (2011) "Prevalence of ADHD and associated features among children in France." *Journal of Attention Disorders 15*, 6, 1516.

Lofthouse, N., Hendren, R., Hurt, E., Arnold, L.E. and Butter, E. (2012) "A Review of Complementary and Alternative Treatments for Autism Spectrum Disorders." Available at www.hindawi.com/journals/aurt/2012/870391, accessed on December 24, 2013.

Lubit, R.H. (2013) "Oppositional Defiant Disorder." Available at http://emedicine.medscape.com/article/918095-overview#aw2aab6b2, accessed on December 24, 2013.

Maglione, M.A., Gans, D., Das, L. *et al.* (2012) "Non-medical interventions for children with ASD." *Pediatrics 130*, Supplement 2, S169–S178.

March, J. and Vitiello, B. (2009) "Clinical messages from the treatment for adolescents with depression study (TADS)." *American Journal Psychiatry* 166, 1118–1123.

McVoy, M. and Findling, R. (2013) *Clinical Manual of Child and Adolescent Psychopharmacology* (2nd edition). Washington, DC: American Psychiatric Publishing.

Miller, I. (2012) "ADHD and sensory modulation disorder: a comparison of behavior and physiology." *Research in Developmental Disabilities 33*, 3, 804.

Mohiuddin, S. (2012) "Psychopharmacology of ASDs: a selective review." *Autism,* August 14.

Murphy, S. (2013) "Deaths: final report for 2010." *National Vital Statistics Reports 61*, 4, 18.

Myers, S. (2007) "Management of children with ASDs." *Pediatrics 120*, 5, 1183.

New Clinical Drug Evaluation Unit 53rd Annual Meeting. Abstract 3. Presented May 29, 2013.

Olfson, M. Ganeroff, M.J., Marcus, S.C. *et al.* (2003) "National trends in the treatment of attention deficit hyperactivity disorder." *American Journal of Psychiatry 160,* 6, 1071–1077.

Osman, B.B. (1997) *Learning Disabilities and ADHD: A Family Guide to Living and Learning Together.* New York: Wiley.

Packer, L. (2005) Tourette Syndrome "Plus." New York: Leslie E. Packer. Available at www.tourettesyndrome.net, accessed on November 13, 2013.

Papolos, D. (2006) *The Bipolar Child.* New York: Broadway Books.

Phelan, T.W. (1994) *Surviving Your Adolescents: How to Manage and Let Go of Your 13–18 Year Olds.* Glen Ellyn, IL: Child Management Press.

Piacentini, J. (2010) "Behavior therapy for children with Tourette disorder: a randomised controlled study." *JAMA: The Journal of the American Medical Association 303*, 19, 1929–1937.

Pontifex, M. (2012) "Exercise improves behavioral, neurocognitive, and scholastic performance in children with ADHD." *The Journal of Pediatrics 162*, 3, 543.

Prasad, V. (2013) "How effective are drug treatments for children with ADHD at improving on-task behavior and academic achievement in the school classroom? A systematic review and meta-analysis." *European Child and Adolescent Psychiatry 22*, 203–216.

Prince, J. and Wilens, T. (2009) "Pharmacotherapy of ADHD and Comorbidities." In T. Brown (ed.) *ADHD Comorbidities: Handbook for ADHD Complications in Children and Adults.* Washington, DC: American Psychiatric Publishing, Inc..

Ratey, J.J. and Johnson, C. (1998) *Shadow Syndromes: The Mild Forms of Mental Disorder That Sabotage Us.* New York: Bantam Books.

Schatschneider, C. and Torgesen, J.K. (2004) "Using our current understanding of dyslexia to support early identification and intervention." *Journal of Child Neurology 19*, 759–765.

Schminky, M. and Baran, J. (1999) "CAPD: an overview of assessment and management practices." *Deaf-Blind Perspectives*, Fall.

Shalev, R. (2004) "Developmental dyscalculia." *Journal of Child Neurology 19*, 10, 765–771.

Shaywitz, S. (2003) *Overcoming Dyslexia: A New and Complete Science-Based Program for Reading Problems at any Level.* New York: Vintage Books.

Shore, K. (2002) *Special Kids Problem Solver: Ready-to-Use Interventions for Helping All Students with Academic, Behavioral, and Physical Problems.* San Francisco, CA: Jossey-Bass.

Shreeram, S. (2009) "Prevalence of eneuresis and its association with ADHD among US children." *Journal of the American Academy of Child and Adolescent Psychiatry 48*, 1, 35–41.

Sonuga-Barke, J. (2013) "Nonpharmaological interventions for ADHD: systematic review and meta-analysis of randomised controlled trials of dietary and psychological treatments." *American Journal Psychiatry 170*, 3, 275.

Strasburger, V. (2011) "Policy statement: children, adolescents, obesity and the media." *Pediatrics 128*, 201–208.

Strawn, J., Patino, R., Schneider, M. *et al.* (2013) "Long-chain omega-3 fatty acids in child and adolescent psychiatry: 1. phenomenonology." *Child and Adolescent Psychopharmacology News 18*, 5, 3.

Szymanski, L.S. and Kaplan, L.C. (2004) "Mental Retardation." In J. Weiner and M. Dulcan (eds) *Textbook of Child and Adolescent Psychiatry* (3rd edition). Arlington, VA: American Psychiatric Publishing.

Tannock R. (2009) "ADHD with Anxiety Disorders." In T. Brown (ed.) *ADHD Comorbidities: Handbook for ADHD Complications in Children and Adults.* Washington: American Psychiatric Publishing, Inc.

Tavernise, S. (2013) "To reduce suicide rates, new focus turns to guns." *New York Times*, February 13.

Thompson, S. (1996) "Non verbal learning disabilities." Available at www.ldonline.org/article/6114.

Torgesen, J. (2004) "Avoiding the devastating downward spiral: the evidence that early intervention prevents reading failure." *American Educator*, Fall, 6–9.

Tourettes Syndrome Study Group. (2002) "Treatment of ADHD in children with tics: a randomised controlled trial." *Neurology 58*, 4, 527.

Waslick, B. and Greenhill, L. (2004) "Attention Deficit/Hyperactivity Disorder." In J. Wiener and M. Dulcan (eds) *Textbook of Child and Adolescent Psychiatry* (3rd edition). Arlington, VA: American Psychiatric Publishing.

Wattenberg, R. (2004) "Waiting rarely works: 'late bloomers' usually just wilt." *American Educator*, Fall, 10–11.

Weller, E., Weller, R., and Danielyan, A. (2004) "Mood Disorders in Prepubertal Children." In J. Wiener and M. Dulcan (eds) *Textbook of Child and Adolescent Psychiatry* (3rd edition). Arlington, VA: American Psychiatric Publishing.

Wiener, J.M. and Dulcan, M.K. (eds) (2004) *Textbook of Child and Adolescent Psychiatry* (3rd edition). Arlington, VA: American Psychiatric Publishing.

Wilens, T.E., Adler, L.A., Adams, J., Sgambati, S., Rotrosen, J., Sawtelle, R., *et al.* (2008). "Misuse and diversion of stimulants prescribed for ADHD: a systematic review of the literature." *Journal of American Academy of Child and Adolescent Psychiatry 47*, 1, 21.

Wilens, T.E., Faraone, S.V., Biederman, J. and Gunawardene, S. (2003) "Does stimulant therapy of attention deficit/hyperactivity disorder beget substance abuse? A meta-analytic review of the literature." *Pediatrics 111*, 11, 179–185.

Willey, L.H. (1999) *Pretending to Be Normal: Living with Asperger's Syndrome.* London: Jessica Kingsley Publishers.

Wu, S. (2010) "Tic suppression: the medical model." *Journal of Child and Adolescent Psychopharmacology 20*, 4, 263.

Zeigler Dendy, C. (2006) *Teenagers with ADD: A Parents' Guide.* Bethesda, MD: Woodbine House.

About the Authors

Martin L. Kutscher, MD is double board certified in Pediatrics and in Neurology, with Special Qualification in Child Neurology. Dr. Kutscher was an Assistant Clinical Professor of Pediatrics and of Neurology at the New York Medical College for more than two decades. He trained at Columbia University's College of Physicians and Surgeons, Temple University's St. Christopher's Hospital for Children, and the Albert Einstein College of Medicine. Dr. Kutscher has more than 25 years of experience diagnosing and treating families affected by ADHD, autism spectrum, LD, tics, and other neurobehavioral disorders. The doctor has lectured internationally on the topics, and has published four other books including: *Organizing the Disorganized Child* (with Marcella Moran); *ADHD—Living without Brakes* (Jessica Kingsley Publishers), and *The ADHD BOOK: Living Right Now!* (Neurology Press). Dr. Kutscher's medical practice is limited to pediatric behavioral neurology, with his main office in Rye Brook, NY. Phone: (914) 232-1810. His website is www.pediatricneurology.com.

Tony Attwood, PhD is recognized as the world's leading authority on Asperger's syndrome. Professor Attwood received an honours degree in psychology from the University of Hull, Master's degree in clinical psychology from the University of Surrey, and PhD from the University of London. Tony is an adjunct professor at Griffith University in Queensland Australia and the senior consultant at the Minds and Hearts clinic for ASD in Brisbane, Australia. Tony wrote the ground-breaking book *Asperger's Syndrome: A Guide for Parents and Professionals* (1998, Jessica Kingsley Publishers), and has published and lectured widely around the world.

Robert R. Wolff, MD is double board certified in Pediatrics and in Neurology with Special Qualification in Child Neurology. Dr. Wolff received his BA from Princeton and his MD from Boston University School of Medicine. He completed a pediatric internship and residency at Yale-New Haven Hospital. His neurology residency and pediatric neurology fellowship were completed at Columbia University's Neurological Institute. He is currently a child neurologist at the Boston Children's Hospital at Waltham, Massachusetts.

Subject Index

Abilify (aripiprazole) 275–6, 278
academic achievement 23
acceptance 27–8
accommodations 24
Adderall 262
ADHD *see* attention deficit hyperactivity
    disorder (ADHD)
affection demonstrations 160–1
affective education 157
agorophobia 176
alexithymia 157
alpha-2 agonists 205, 238, 277
amphetamines 262–3
anger
    in ADHD 62–3
    in Asperger's syndrome 143
    avoidance of 30
    calming techniques 46–51
    quiz 51–2
anti-bullying programs 156
anticonvulsants 274–5
antidepressants 215, 272–3
anxiety disorders 171–6
    cf. normal childhood concerns 172–3
    co-morbidities 17–18, 236
    incidence and prevalence 13, 172
    medications 272–3
    neurological basis 172
appetite problems 211
Applied Behavioral Analysis (ABA)
    135–6
arguments 42–3, 47, 64, 231–4
arrogance 143

Asperger's syndrome 123–4, 137–69
    characteristics 142–4
    classification 137–9
    diagnosis 127
    gender difference 140–1
    identifying strengths and weaknesses
        144–6
    learning abilities and styles 161–3
    long-term outlook 169
    managing emotions 156161
    medication use 160
    special interests 163–9
    treatment programs 147–56
    see also high-functioning autism
assignments 70–4
    incomplete 73–4
    marking 73–4
Ativan (lorazepam) 273
attention deficit hyperactivity disorder
    (ADHD)
    co-morbidities and clusters 17–19,
        64–6, 235–6, 245–6
    definitions 53–9
    first signs 19–22
    formal evaluations 23–4
    incidence 13
    neurological basis 66–7
    prevalence 66
    problem magnitude 13–14, 78–80
    symptoms 59–64
    treatment principles 27–52, 68–78
        comparative effectiveness 268–9
        medications 76–7, 182, 258–69
        non-pharmacological 77–8

attention difficulties 63
Attributes Activity 144–6
auditory processing skills 242–3
autism spectrum disorder (ASD) 111–36
    classification of conditions 121–35
        expanded disorders 125–30
    co-morbidities 17–18
    communication difficulties 112–19
    incidence 13
    level 1 (Asperger's syndrome) 137–69
    treatments 135–6
        medications 277–9
autistic disorder 122
    see also autism spectrum disorder
        (ASD)

basal ganglia 67
behavior change strategies 36–52
    see also cognitive behavioral therapy
        (CBT)
behavior management training 50
behavioral checklist 281–2
behavioral explosions 239–40
    see also anger; temper outbursts
benzodiazepines 273
bipolar disorders 209–10, 219–30
    characteristics and symptoms 220–4
    co-morbidities 18, 223, 230
    definitions and classifications 210,
        219–24
    importance of communication 227–8
    medications 230, 274–6
    school support 225–30
    see also depression
blame, avoidance of 28–9, 32, 43
blaming others 64
body language 113–14, 118
brain function 34
    in ADHD 66–7
    in anxiety disorders 172
    in depression 214
    in SID 183–4
    in Tourette's/tics 200
    neural plasticity 190
    stress responses 46
brainstem auditory evoked responses
        (BAER) 247
bribes 39
buddies 153

bullying, school policies 156
Buspar (busipirone) 273

calendars and planners 70
calming techniques 15, 46–51, 194
care plans and accommodations 24
caregivers, adjusting own behaviors
        27–33, 41
Catapres (clonidine) 205, 238, 267–8,
        277
catatonia 139
Celexa (citalopram) 270–1, 271
central auditory processing (CAP) 112
central auditory processing (CAP)
        disorder 241–52
    co-morbidities 18
    definitions and classifications 241246
    diagnosis and tests 246–7
    support and adaptations 248–52
changing behaviors
    caregivers 27–33, 41
    children 36–52
childhood disintegrative disorder 125
children with ADHD
    mindsets and perspectives 33–6
    understanding their perceptions 33–6
classification of conditions (general
        principles) 12–13
classroom management, general
        principles 51
cleaning obsessions 178
clusters of conditions see "syndrome mix"
co-morbidities (overview) 11, 17–19
"coddling" children 30
cognitive behavioral therapy (CBT)
    for Asperger's syndrome 156, 160–1
    for depression 214–15
    for OCD 181–2
cognitive restructuring 157
collaborative problem-solving techniques
        (Greene 2010) 49–50
communication
    classification of disorders 120–35
    skills needed 112–19
    teacher-parent 32, 70, 71–3, 227–8
    theories 114–15
comprehension problems 95
Comprehensive Behavioral Intervention
        for Tics (CIBT) 204–5

compulsions 177
computer games 153
  limiting play 76, 237–8
concentration problems 211
Concerta 260
conduct disorder 88, 233
  see also oppositional defiant disorder
    (ODD)
conversation skills 155–6
cooling off periods 48–9
coprolalia 198
counseling, for depression 214–15
creativity 101
cursing 64, 198

Daytrana Patch 261
decoding (reading) 93–5, 96
defusion techniques 46–9
Depakote (sodium valproate) 238, 274,
    275
depression 207–17
  co-morbidities 18, 142, 236
  common symptoms 210–13
  definitions and classifications 207–10
  incidence 13
  medications 215–16, 269–72
  neurological basis 214
  school-based support 216–17
  therapies 214–15, 216
depressive episodes, coping strategies
    216–17, 229
desensitization therapies 192
developmental coordination disorder
    85–6
Dexedrine 262
dextro-amphetamine preparations 262
diagnosis 17–25
  classification systems 12–13
  co-morbidities 17–19
  early signs 19–22
  formal evaluations 23–4
  see also individual conditions
*Diagnostic and Statistical Manual of
    Mental Disorders (DSM)* 12–13
  ADHD 53–5
  anxiety disorders 171, 175
  ASDs 121–35
  Asperger's syndrome 137–9
  bipolar disorder 219–22

depression and dysthymia 207–10
  intellectual disability 108–9
  intermittent explosive disorder 239
  language disorder 112–13
  learning disorders 83–5
  oppositional defiant disorder (ODD)
    231–3
"disability outlook" 28–9
discrimination (noise) 242
disorganization 54–5, 61
  treatments and support 68–76
disruptive mood dysregulation disorder
    (DMDD) 208–9
distractibility 54, 220
dopamine 46, 67, 200, 258, 266–7
drama classes 153–4
driving accidents 259
dyscalculia 104–6
dysgraphia 85–6, 106–7
dyslexia 92–104
  acting out behaviors 34
  condition characteristics 92–5
  early detection and treatments 95–104
  school accommodations 101–2
  specialized instruction programs 102–4
  strengths 101
  teacher/parent-led programs 98–101
dysthymia 208
  see also depression

educational tests 23
  see also assignments
"effective independence" 31–2
Effexor (venlafaxine) 272
Elavil (amitriptyline) 215, 270–1, 272
emotional reactions
  in ADHD 58–9
  in Asperger's syndrome 142–4
Emotional Toolbox (Attwood) 154,
    157–8
emotions, management of 156–61
empathy 114–15, 121–2, 130, 202, 233
enticements 39
euphoria 220
evaluations and screening 23–4, 190–1
exams and classroom tests, coping
    strategies 163
executive function 56–9
  quiz 285–7

exercise, making time for 69
explosive behaviors 239–40
    see also anger; temper outbursts
Exposure and Response Prevention
    (ERP) 181
expressive verbal language 112–13
externalization, of thoughts and feelings
    143–4
eye contact 68, 118

failures
    forgiveness of 33
    personal responsibility for 32–3
family stress 211
fears
    normal childhood concerns 172–3
    see also anxiety disorders
feedback giving 39, 155
    on medication effectiveness 228
feelings, internalization of 142–3
fights, defusion techniques 46–9
figure-ground 242
fine motor skills 126, 189
    therapies 196
firearms 213–14
fish oils 78, 215, 269, 274, 277
Focalin (dexmethylphenidate) 260
Focalin XR 261
foresight 56–7, 59–60
"four cardinal sins" (Phelan 1994) 42
freezing (movements) 139
friendships
    child–adult relations 149
    difficulties in forming 63
    programs 148–55
    romantic 148
    stages of 147–56
    therapy suggestions 155–6
frustration feelings 30, 62
fun and laughter 36

GAD *see* generalized anxiety disorder
    (GAD)
gender difference, Asperger's syndrome
    140–1
generalized anxiety disorder (GAD)
    171–5
genetics 18
    of ADHD 67
    of OCD/anxiety disorders/tics 200

goal setting 40
    difficulties 64
grandiose thinking 220
gross motor skills 126
guidelines for treatment 27–36
    adjusting own mindset 27–33
    children's perspectives 33–6
guns 213–14

Habit Reversal Training (HRT) 204–5
Haldol (haloperidal) 275–6, 277
hallucinations 223, 271
handwriting problems *see* dysgraphia
hearing tests 246–8
helping too much 30
high-functioning autism 125
    see also Asperger's syndrome
hindsight 57, 60
homework *see* school assignments
hyper-focusing 62
hyper-responsiveness 63
hyperactivity difficulties, in ADHD 54–5
hyperlexia 129
hypersensitivity 185–6
hypomanic episodes 221
hyposensitivity 186

imagination, internalization of 142–3
imitation 143–4
    in Asperger's syndrome 143–4
incidence of ADHD 13
inconsistent behaviors 62
independence issues 31–2
inflexibility 63
inhibition 55–6
insomnia, coping strategies 289–90
intellectual disability 107–10
intelligence 81–2, 108–9
interactive computer games 153
interests
    loss of 210
    see also special interests
intermittent explosive disorder 210,
    239–40
internalization
    of rules 62
    of thoughts and feelings 142–3
Internet
    as learning aid 91–2, 102
    limiting screen time 76, 237–8
    social media 155

intervention (general guidance)
  fears of over-protection 30
  providing "safety nets" 31
  teaching independence 31–2
  timing of 44
  see also treatment principles
Intuniv 267–8
IQ (Intelligence Quotient) 81–2, 108–9
irritability
  long lasting 224
  severe 207–9, 211, 220

"joint attention" 117–18
"just stop!" 48–9

Kapvay 267–8
Klonopin (clonazepam) 273

labeling 126
Lamictal (lamotrigine) 238, 275
language skills 112–13, 115–16
laughter and humor 36
learning disorders (LDs)
  co-morbidities 17–18, 64–5
  definitions 82–6
  early signs 86–7
  general support 88–9
  homework 89–90
  impact 87–8
  prevalence 83
  reading difficulties 92–104
  specialized programs 102–4
  use of technology 91–2, 102
learning styles 161–3
Lexapro (escitalopram) 215, 270–1
limbic system 67, 184
lithium 275
Live Scribe pen 102
living in the present 60–1
localization (noise) 242
love 28
Luvox (Fluvoxamine) 271
lying 64

major depressive episodes 208, 210, 221
manic episodes 209–10, 220–1
  coping strategies 228–9
mathematics disorder 104–6
medical evaluations 23–4

medications 258–79
  attitudes towards 256
  benefits 254
  concerns 254–5
  dependency issues 255–6
  evaluation and feedback 228
  for ADHD 76–7, 182, 258–69
    comparative effectiveness 268–9
    side effects 263–6, 267–8
  for anxiety 272–3
  for autism spectrum disorders (ASD)
    277–9
  for bipolar disorder 274–6
  for depression 215–16, 269–72
    side effects 270–1
  for OCD 182, 274
  for tic disorders 276–7
  prescribing 256–8
  side effects 263–6, 270–1, 272–3
  and substance abuse 255
meltdowns, defusion techniques 46–9
memory, in ADHD 57–8, 60
mental health problems, rates of 13
mental retardation *see* intellectual
  disability
Metadate CD 261
methylphenidate preparations 259–61
"mirror traits" 37–8
mistakes 162
mood disorders, classification of 207–10
mood stabilizers 238, 274–5
motivation 39–40
  encouragement of 162
motor skills 126
  fine 126, 189, 196
  gross 126
mutism 175

nagging 42
negative reinforcement 40
negative tones and emotions 35, 236
negotiating techniques, using
  collaborative problem-solving 49–50
neural plasticity 190
neuroleptics 206, 238, 275–6
neurological findings *see* brain function
neurotransmitters 214
nightmares 223
"no-fault approach" (Zeigler Dendy
  2006) 42–3

non-verbal communication 113–14, 118
skill deficits 126–7
non-verbal learning disabilities (NVLD/
NLD) 125–7
norepinephrine 214
notebooks 70
NVLD *see* non-verbal learning
disabilities (NVLD/NLD)

obscenities 198
obsessions 177
see also obsessive-compulsive disorder
(OCD); special interests
obsessive-compulsive disorder (OCD)
177–82
co-morbidities 17–18
professional treatments 181–2
medications 274
school-based treatments 178–81
omega-3/omega-6 78, 215, 269, 274, 277
"one-track" mind 163
oppositional defiant disorder (ODD)
231–40
co-morbidities 18, 235–6
definitions and classifications 231–2,
240
incidence and impact 234–5
medications 238
support measures and treatments
236–8
Orap (pimozide) 275–6, 277
organization problems 58, 61
treatments and support 68–76
over-protection fears 30–1
ownership and responsibilities 32

Pamelor 215
PANDAS 201
panic disorder 176
paperwork organization 70
parents, adjusting own behaviors 27–33
Paxil (paroxetine) 271
PDD-NOS (PDD-not otherwise
specified) 124
PDDs *see* pervasive development
disorders (PDDs)
peer group acceptance 152
perfectionism 173
persistent depressive disorder *see*
dysthymia

pervasive development disorders (PDDs)
121–2
Phelan's "four cardinal sins" 42
phenomes 93–4
phobias 175–6
phonics 98, 103
planners *see* schedules and planners
planning problems 58
see also disorganization
plasticity (neural) 190
play skills 117, 147–8
see also friendships
positive feedback 155
positive reinforcement 38–40
positivity 36–45, 237
Post-it notes 69
pragmatic language 115–16
priapism 265
problem-solving difficulties 58
problem-solving techniques, collaborative
approaches 49–50
proprioceptive sense 184
therapies 195
prospective memory 57
Prozac (fluxetine) 182, 215, 271, 278
psycho-educational tests 23
psychological tests 23
punishments 38, 41–2, 44–5
legal perspectives 44, 227

Quillivant 261

racing speech 220
Raising Resilient Children (Brooks and
Goldstein) 27–8
reading disorders *see* dyslexia; hyperlexia
reading process 93–5
reading programs 102–4
reading support 98–101
rebound 263–4
receptive verbal language 112
relationships in adolescence 148
see also friendships
relaxation tools 15
resentment feelings 40–1
coping strategies 41–5
Rett's syndrome 124
reward systems 36–7, 38–9
risk-seeking behaviors 224

Risperdal (risperidone) 206, 238, 275–6, 277–8
Ritalin 259–60, 278
Ritalin RA 261
ritualistic behaviors 118–19
rituals 175, 178–81
romantic relations 148
rules of social engagement 116

sadness feelings 210
"safety nets" 31
schedules and planners 70–1
school assignments 70–4
    incomplete 73–4
school-home communication 32, 70, 71–3
schoolwork supplies 70
screen time, limiting 76, 237–8
screening 190–1
seating arrangements 68, 248
selective mutism 175
self-awareness problems 61
self-esteem problems 210, 220
self-harm 178, 212–13
self-help guides 154
self-regulation, of/by emotions 59
self-talk 57
semantic language 112–13
semantic-pragmatic language disorder (SPLD) 128–9
sensory discrimination problems 187
sensory integration dysfunction (SID/SPD) 183–96
    co-morbidities 18, 189
    common symptoms 187–9
    diagnosis and evaluation 190–2
    long-term outlook 196
    neurological basis 183–4
    support and treatments 189–90, 191–6
sensory modulation problems 187
sensory-based motor problems 187
separation anxiety 175
serotonin 214
signs and symptoms (overview) 19–22
sleep problems
    anxiety disorders 174–5
    depression 211
    manic episodes 220
    support measures 289–90
social anxiety disorder 176

social documentaries 150–5
social engineering 152
social skill deficits
    in ADHD 62
    in ASD 113–22, 147–56
    categories and classification 120–35
Social Stories™ 150–2
socialization skills 113–14
spatial orientation skills 126
special interests 118, 163–9
    causes 165–6
    during adolescence 165
    as emotional restorative 159
    and friendships 168–9
    gender differences 164–5
    modifying behaviors 166–8
    rewards and motivation 167–8
    ritualistic behaviors 118
specific learning disorders (LDs) see learning disorders (LDs)
specific phobia 175
speech tests 247–8
SSRIs (selective serotonin reuptake inhibitors) 182, 215–16, 270–1, 272
    side effects 270–1
stalking behaviors 165
stealing 64
sticker charts 38–9
stimulants 258–66
    side effects 263–6
Strattera (atomoxetine) 267, 277–8
strengths and weaknesses 36–8
    identification activities 144–6
stress
    on families 211
    on teachers 212
stress responses
    brain functions 46
    in children 34
"stress speedometer" 47–8
substance abuse 88
suicide 212–13
    prevention 213–14
support groups 154
swearing 64
symbolic play 117, 127
"syndrome mix" 17–19

taboo thoughts 178
taboo words 198

tactile sense 183–4
  therapies 194–5
tantrums
  severe 207–10
  see also temper outbursts
teachers
  communication issues 32
  importance 32
teamwork skills 153
teen behaviors 35–6
  and Asperger's syndrome 144, 148,
    152–6
teen interests 165
"Teflon syndrome" 87
Tegretol (carbamazepine) 238, 275
temper outbursts
  extreme 223, 224, 239–40
  short-lived 62–3
temporal patterning tests 247–8
Tenex (guanfacine) 205, 238, 267–8, 277
theory of mind 114–15
thoughts
  taboos 178
  unwanted 178
thrill-seeking behaviors 63
tics 178, 197–206
  classification 197–8
  incidence 199–200
  long-term outlook 200–1
  medications 205–6, 264, 276–7
  professional therapies 204–5
  school-based treatments 201–20
  self-control 201
time awareness problems 58, 61
time out techniques 48–9
timing of responses 44
Tofranil 215
token systems 36–7, 38–9
Tourette's syndrome 198–200
  co-morbidities 17–18
  incidence 13
  see also tics
transitioning difficulties 58, 62
treatment principles 27–52
  general guidelines 27–36
  rules for behavior change 36–51
tricyclic antidepressants 215, 272–3
  side effects 272–3

unspecified anxiety disorder 176
unwritten rules 116

Valium (diazepam) 273
verbalization learning styles 161–2
vestibular sense 184
  therapies 195
video recordings 150
visual exercises 94
visualization learning styles 161–2
vocal tics 198
Vyvanse (lisdexamfetamine) 262

Wechsler Intelligence Scale for Children
    (WISC) 23, 81–2, 108
weight gain, medication side effects 274,
    275
Wellbutrin (bupropion) 268
Weschler Individual Achievement Test
    (WIAT) 23
word lists 99
word processors 91
working memory 57
worries, normal childhood concerns
    172–3
written expression disorder 106–7

Xanax (alprazolam) 273

Zoloft (setraline) 271
Zyprexa (olanzepine) 275–6

Author Index

AACAP 213
American Academy of Pediatrics (AAP) 191–2, 237, 278
American Occupational Therapy Association (AOTA) 190
American Psychiatric Association (APA) 83–4, 85–6, 123, 132, 134, 136, 137, 169, 171, 178, 207–9, 221–2, 239–40
Arnstein, A. 46

Bader, A. 78
Baeyens, D. 67
Baran, J. 242
Barkley, R.A. 28–9, 33, 36, 38–9, 55–7, 62–4, 67, 74, 231
Beiderman, J. 259
Bernstein, G. 172, 174
Biederman, J. 79
Bloch, M. 78, 267, 269
Brent, D.A. 213
Brooks, R. 27–8, 35, 37
Brown, T. 50, 56, 59

Carver, J. 41–2
CDC 11, 13, 213
Chandler, J. 237
Charach, A. 68
Covey, S.R. 47

Danielyan, A. 217, 230

Feinstein, C. 83, 88, 93, 107
Findling, R. 233

Florida Department of Education 248
Freeman, J.B. 274

Gabbay, V. 277
Garnett, K. 104–6
Goldstein, S. 27–8, 35, 37, 255, 274
Greene, R.W. 38–40, 46–7, 49–50, 63, 232
Greenhill, L. 199

Hallowell, E. 28, 31, 37–8
Hammerness, P. 265
Harris, E. 199
Hodgeson, K. 269
Houston, A. 13

Jensen, P. 28, 31, 37–8, 76
Johnson, C. 19

Kaplan, L.C. 108
King, R. 199–200
Klein, R. 78–9
Kranowitz, C.S. 185, 190, 193–6
Kutscher, M.L. 56, 65–6, 76, 107

Larson, K. 18, 64–5
Layne, A. 172, 174
Leckman, J. 199–200
Lofthouse, N. 279
Lubit, R.H. 234–5

McVoy, M. 233
Maglione, M.A. 136

March, J. 216
Miller, I. 192
Mohiuddin, S. 277
Moran, M. 76, 107
Murphy, S. 213
Myers, S. 135

New Clinical Drug Evaluation Unit 65

Olfson, M. 66
Osman, B.B. 82, 86, 89–90

Packer, L. 179–81, 199, 202–4
Papolos, D. 223
Phelan, T.W. 42
Phillips, I. 83, 88, 93, 107
Piacentini, J. 205
Pontifex, M. 69
Prasad, V. 259
Prince, J. 199, 266

Qawasmi, A. 78, 269

Ratey, J.J. 19

Schatschneider, C. 96
Schminky, M. 242
Shalev, R. 104
Shaywitz, S. 94–5, 96–8, 101–4
Shore, K. 98–101, 173, 179
Shreeram, S. 67
Sonuga-Barke, J. 78
Strasburger, V. 76
Strawn, J. 215, 274
Szymanski, L.S. 108

Tannock, R. 175, 182, 265, 267
Tavernise, S. 213
Thompson, S. 125–6
Torgesen, J. 95–6

Vitiello, B. 216

Waslick, B. 199
Wattenberg, R. 95–6
Weller, E. 217, 230
Weller, R. 217, 230
Wilens, T. 199, 255, 266

Willey, L.H. 29, 36, 116, 119
Wu, S. 199, 277

Zeigler Dendy, C. 42–3

Barclay Public Library
220 South Main Street
PO Box 349
Warrensburg, IL 62573